Contents

Treatment of tuberculosis
GUIDELINES

Fourth edition

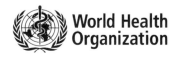

World Health Organization

WHO Library Cataloguing-in-Publication Data:

Treatment of tuberculosis: guidelines – 4th ed.

WHO/HTM/TB/2009.420

1.Antitubercular agents – administration and dosage. 2.Tuberculosis,
Pulmonary – drug therapy. 3.National health programs. 4.Patient compliance.
5.Guidelines. I.World Health Organization. Stop TB Dept.

ISBN 978 92 4 154783 3   (NLM classification: WF 360)

Designed by minimum graphics
Printed in Italy by La Tipografica Varese S.p.A., Varese

Abbreviations

AFB	acid-fast bacilli
AIDS	acquired immunodeficiency syndrome
ART	antiretroviral therapy
DOT	directly observed treatment
DOTS	the internationally agreed strategy for TB control
DRS	drug resistance surveillance
DST	drug susceptibility testing
E	ethambutol
EPTB	extrapulmonary tuberculosis
EQA	external quality assurance
FDC	fixed-dose combination
GLC	Green Light Committee
H	isoniazid
HIV	human immunodeficiency virus
ISTC	International Standards for Tuberculosis Care
MDR	multidrug resistance
MDR-TB	multidrug-resistant tuberculosis
NNRTI	non-nucleoside reverse transcriptase inhibitor
NRTI	nucleoside reverse transcriptase inhibitor
NTP	national tuberculosis control programme
PTB	pulmonary tuberculosis
R	rifampicin
S	streptomycin
TB	tuberculosis
TB/HIV	HIV-related TB
XDR-TB	extensively drug-resistant tuberculosis
Z	pyrazinamide

Acknowledgements

The Stop TB Department of the World Health Organization gratefully acknowledges the members of the Guidelines Group (listed in Annex 6), including Jeremiah Muhwa Chakaya, the Chairperson.

Richard Menzies (McGill University, Montreal, Canada), Karen Steingart and Phillip Hopewell (University of California, San Francisco, USA) and Andrew Nunn and Patrick Phillips (British Medical Research Council) led the teams that compiled, synthesized and evaluated the evidence underlying each recommendation.

Suzanne Hill and Holger Schünemann facilitated the meeting of the Guidelines Group.

Useful feedback was obtained from the External Review Group (also listed in Annex 6) and from WHO and UNAIDS staff.

Additional feedback and support were provided by the Guidelines Review Committee (Chair, Suzanne Hill; Secretariat, Faith McLellan).

Publication of the guidelines was supported in part by a financial contribution from the Global Fund to Fight AIDS, Tuberculosis and Malaria.

The document was prepared by Sarah Royce and Malgorzata Grzemska.

Dorris Ortega provided secretarial support.

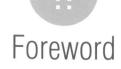

Foreword

The World Health Organization's Stop TB Department has prepared this fourth edition of *Treatment of tuberculosis: guidelines*, adhering fully to the new WHO process for evidence-based guidelines. Several important recommendations are being promoted in this new edition.

First, the recommendation to discontinue the regimen based on just 2 months of rifampicin (2HRZE/6HE) and change to the regimen based on a full 6 months of rifampicin (2HRZE/4HR) will reduce the number of relapses and failures. This will alleviate patient suffering resulting from a second episode of tuberculosis (TB) and conserve patient and programme resources.

Second, this fourth edition confirms prior WHO recommendations for drug susceptibility testing (DST) at the start of therapy for all previously treated patients. Finding and treating multidrug-resistant TB (MDR-TB) in previously treated patients will help to improve the very poor outcomes in these patients. New recommendations for the prompt detection and appropriate treatment of (MDR-TB) cases will also improve access to life-saving care. The retreatment regimen with first-line drugs (formerly called "Category 2" regimen) is ineffective in MDR-TB; it is therefore critical to detect MDR-TB promptly so that an effective regimen can be started.

Third, detecting MDR-TB will require expansion of DST capacity within the context of country-specific, comprehensive plans for laboratory strengthening. This fourth edition provides guidance for treatment approaches in the light of advances in laboratory technology and the country's progress in building laboratory capacity. In countries that use the new rapid molecular-based tests, DST results for rifampicin/isoniazid will be available within 1–2 days and can be used in deciding which regimen should be started for the individual patient. Rapid tests eliminate the need to treat "in the dark" during the long wait for results of DST by other methods (weeks for liquid media methods or months for solid media methods).

Because of the delays in obtaining results, this new edition recommends that countries using conventional DST methods should start treatment with an empirical regimen. If there is a high likelihood of MDR-TB, empirical treatment with an MDR regimen is recommended until DST results are available. Drug resistance surveillance (DRS) data or surveys will be required to identify subgroups of TB patients with the highest prevalence of MDR-TB, such as those whose prior treatment has failed. Implementation of these recommendations will require every country to include an MDR-TB regimen in its standards for treatment in collaboration with the Green Light Committee Initiative.

Fourth, diagnosing MDR-TB cases among previously treated patients and providing effective treatment will greatly help in halting the *spread* of MDR-TB. This edition also addresses the prevention of *acquired* MDR-TB, especially among new TB patients who already have isoniazid-resistant *Mycobacterium tuberculosis* when they start treatment. The meta-analyses that form the evidence base for this revision revealed that new patients with isoniazid-resistant TB have a greatly increased risk of acquiring additional drug resistance. To prevent amplification of existing drug resistance, this edition includes the option of adding ethambutol to the continuation phase of treatment for new patients in populations with high prevalence of isoniazid resistance. In addition, the daily dosing recommended for the intensive phase may also help in reducing acquired drug resistance, especially in patients with pretreatment isoniazid resistance.

Finally, this edition strongly reaffirms prior recommendations for supervised treatment, as well as the use of fixed-dose combinations of anti-TB drugs and patient kits as further measures for preventing the acquisition of drug resistance.

Use of the new WHO process for evidence-based guidelines revealed many key unanswered questions. What is the best way to treat isoniazid-resistant TB and prevent MDR? What is the optimal duration of TB treatment in HIV-positive patients? Which patients are most likely to relapse and how can they be detected and treated? Identification of such crucial questions for the future research agenda is an important outcome of this revision and will require careful follow-up to ensure that answers will be provided to further strengthen TB care practices.

As new studies help to fill these gaps in knowledge, new laboratory technology is introduced, and new drugs are discovered, these guidelines will be updated and revised. In the meantime, WHO pledges its full support to helping countries to implement and evaluate this fourth edition of *Treatment of tuberculosis: guidelines* and to use the lessons learnt to improve access to high-quality, life-saving TB care.

Dr Mario Raviglione
Director
Stop TB Department

Executive summary

Major progress in global tuberculosis (TB) control followed the widespread implementation of the DOTS strategy. The Stop TB Strategy, launched in 2006, builds upon and enhances the achievements of DOTS. New objectives include universal access to patient-centred treatment and protection of populations from TB/HIV and multidrug-resistant TB (MDR-TB). The Stop TB Strategy and the Global Plan to implement the new strategy make it necessary to revise the third edition of *Treatment of tuberculosis: guidelines for national programmes*, published in 2003.

Creation of the fourth edition follows new WHO procedures for guidelines development. With input from a group of external experts – the Guidelines Group – WHO identified seven key questions, and systematic reviews were conducted for each question. The Guidelines Group based its recommendations on the quality of the evidence (assessed according to the GRADE methodology), patient values, and costs, as well judgements about trade-offs between benefits and harms. Recommendations were rated as "strong" or "conditional".

The evidence and considerations underlying each recommendation are summarized in Annex 2.

A *strong recommendation* is one for which desirable effects of adherence to the recommendation clearly outweigh the undesirable effects. The strong recommendations in this edition use the words "should" or "should not". No alternatives are listed.

A *conditional recommendation* is one for which the desirable effects of adherence to the recommendation probably outweigh the undesirable effects but the trade-offs are uncertain.

Reasons for uncertainty can include:

— lack of high-quality evidence to support the recommendation;
— limited benefits of implementing the recommendation;
— costs not justified by the benefits;
— imprecise estimates of benefit.

A *weak recommendation* is one for which there is insufficient evidence and it is based on field application and expert opinion. Recommendations for which the quality of evidence was not assessed in line with the GRADE methodology are not rated.

Conditional and weak recommendations use the words "may". For several of the conditional recommendations, alternatives are listed.

The recommendations that address each of the seven questions are listed below, and also appear in bold text in Chapter 3 (Standard treatment regimens), Chapter 4 (Monitoring during treatment) and Chapter 5 (Co-management of HIV and active TB). Areas outside the scope of the seven questions, as well as the remaining chapters, have been updated with current WHO TB policies and recent references but were not the subject of systematic literature reviews or of new recommendations by the Guidelines Group.

Question 1. Duration of rifampicin in new patients

Should new pulmonary TB patients be treated with the 6-month rifampicin regimen (2HRZE/4HR) or the 2-month rifampicin regimen (2HRZE/6HE)?

■ Recommendation 1.1

New patients with pulmonary TB should receive a regimen containing 6 months of rifampicin: 2HRZE/4HR

(Strong/High grade of evidence)

Remark a: Recommendation 1.1 also applies to extrapulmonary TB, except TB of the central nervous system, bone or joint for which some expert groups suggest longer therapy (see Chapter 8).

Remark b: WHO recommends that national TB control programmes ensure that supervision and support are provided for all TB patients in order to achieve completion of the full course of therapy.

Remark c: WHO recommends drug resistance surveys (or surveillance) for monitoring the impact of the treatment programme as well as for designing standard regimens.

■ Recommendation 1.2

The 2HRZE/6HE treatment regimen should be phased out

(Strong/High grade of evidence)

Question 2. Dosing frequency in new patients

When a country selects 2HRZE/4HR, should patients be treated with a daily or three times weekly intensive phase?

■ Recommendation 2.1

Wherever feasible, the optimal dosing frequency for new patients with pulmonary TB is daily throughout the course of therapy

(Strong/High grade of evidence)

There are two alternatives to Recommendation 2.1:

■ **Recommendation 2.1A**
New patients with pulmonary TB may receive a daily intensive phase followed by a three times weekly continuation phase [2HRZE/4(HR)$_3$], provided that each dose is directly observed

(Conditional/High and moderate grade of evidence)

■ **Recommendation 2.1B**
Three times weekly dosing throughout therapy [2(HRZE)$_3$/4(HR)$_3$] may be used as another alternative to Recommendation 2.1, provided that every dose is directly observed and the patient is NOT living with HIV or living in an HIV-prevalent setting

(Conditional/High and moderate grade of evidence)

Remark a: Treatment regimens for TB patients living with HIV or living in HIV-prevalent settings are discussed in Recommendation 4 and Chapter 5.

Remark b: In terms of dosing frequency for HIV-negative patients, the systematic review found little evidence of differences in failure or relapse rates with daily or three times weekly regimens (see Annex 2). However, rates of acquired drug resistance were higher among patients receiving three times weekly dosing throughout therapy than among patients who received daily drug administration throughout treatment. Moreover, in patients with pretreatment isoniazid resistance, three times weekly dosing during the intensive phase was associated with significantly higher risks of failure and acquired drug resistance than daily dosing during the intensive phase.

■ **Recommendation 2.2**
New patients with TB should not receive twice weekly dosing for the full course of treatment unless this is done in the context of formal research

(Strong/High grade of evidence)

Remark: The available evidence showed equivalent efficacy of daily intensive-phase dosing followed by two times weekly continuation phase. However, twice weekly dosing is not recommended on operational grounds, since missing one dose means the patient receives only half the regimen.

Question 3. Initial regimen in countries with high levels of isoniazid resistance

In countries with high levels of isoniazid resistance in new TB patients, should the continuation phase (containing isoniazid and rifampicin) be changed in the standard treatment of all new patients, in order to prevent the development of multidrug resistance?[1]

---

[1] This question applies to countries where isoniazid susceptibility testing in new patients is not done (or results are not available) before the continuation phase begins.

■ **Recommendation 3**

In populations with known or suspected high levels of isoniazid resistance, new TB patients may receive HRE as therapy in the continuation phase as an acceptable alternative to HR

(Weak/Insufficient evidence, expert opinion)

Remark a: While there is a pressing need to prevent multidrug resistance (MDR), the most effective regimen for the treatment of isoniazid-resistant TB is not known. There is inadequate evidence to quantify the ability of ethambutol to "protect rifampicin" in patients with pretreatment isoniazid resistance. The evidence for ocular toxicity from ethambutol was not systematically reviewed for this revision, but the risk of permanent blindness exists. Thus, further research (see Annex 5) is urgently needed to define the level of isoniazid resistance that would warrant the addition of ethambutol (or other drugs) to the continuation phase of the standard new patient regimen in TB programmes where isoniazid drug susceptibility testing is not done (or results are unavailable) before the continuation phase begins.

Remark b: Daily (rather than three times weekly) intensive-phase dosing may also help prevent acquired drug resistance in TB patients starting treatment with isoniazid resistance. The systematic review (Annex 2) found that patients with isoniazid resistance treated with a three times weekly intensive phase had significantly higher risks of failure and acquired drug resistance than those treated with daily dosing during the intensive phase.

Question 4. TB treatment in persons living with HIV

Should intermittent regimens be used for persons living with HIV? What should be the duration of TB treatment in people living with HIV?

Remark: Current WHO recommendations promoting the use of antiretroviral therapy in TB patients living with HIV should be put rapidly into practice.

■ **Recommendation 4.1**

TB patients with known positive HIV status and all TB patients living in HIV-prevalent settings should receive daily TB treatment at least during the intensive phase

(Strong/High grade of evidence)

Remark: HIV-prevalent settings are defined as countries, subnational administrative units, or selected facilities where the HIV prevalence among adult pregnant women is ≥1% or among TB patients is ≥5%.

■ **Recommendation 4.2**

For the continuation phase, the optimal dosing frequency is also daily for these patients

(Strong/High grade of evidence)

■ **Recommendation 4.3**

If a daily continuation phase is not possible for these patients, three times weekly dosing during the continuation phase is an acceptable alternative

(Conditional/High and moderate grade of evidence)

■ **Recommendation 4.4**

It is recommended that TB patients who are living with HIV should receive at least the same duration of TB treatment as HIV-negative TB patients

(Strong/High grade of evidence)

Remark a: Some experts recommend prolonging TB treatment in persons living with HIV (see Chapter 5).

Remark b: Previously treated TB patients who are living with HIV should receive the same retreatment regimens as HIV-negative TB patients.

Recommendations 1–4 (as they relate to new patients) are summarized in Table A below, and shown in Tables 3.2 and 3.3 in Chapter 3.

Table A STANDARD REGIMEN AND DOSING FREQUENCY FOR NEW TB PATIENTS

Intensive phase	Continuation phase	Comments
2 months of HRZE[a]	4 months of HR	
2 months of HRZE	4 months of HRE	Applies only in countries with high levels of isoniazid resistance in new TB patients, and where isoniazid drug susceptibility testing in new patients is not done (or results are unavailable) before the continuation phase begins

[a] WHO no longer recommends omission of ethambutol during the intensive phase of treatment for patients with non-cavitary, smear-negative pulmonary TB or extrapulmonary disease who are known to be HIV-negative.

Dosing frequency		Comments
Intensive phase	Continuation phase	
Daily	Daily	Optimal
Daily	3 times per week	Acceptable alternative for any new TB patient receiving directly observed therapy
3 times per week	3 times per week	Acceptable alternative provided that the patient is receiving directly observed therapy and is NOT living with HIV or living in an HIV-prevalent setting (see Chapter 5)

Note: Daily (rather than three times weekly) intensive-phase dosing may help to prevent acquired drug resistance in TB patients starting treatment with isoniazid resistance (see Annex 2).

Question 5. Sputum monitoring during TB treatment of smear-positive pulmonary TB patients

In pulmonary TB patients who are initially smear positive, how effective is monitoring sputum specimens for predicting relapse, failure and pretreatment isoniazid resistance?

Figures 4.1 and 4.2 in Chapter 4 illustrate Recommendations 5.1–5.3.

■ **Recommendation 5.1**

For smear-positive pulmonary TB patients treated with first-line drugs, sputum smear microscopy may be performed at completion of the intensive phase of treatment

(Conditional/High and moderate grade of evidence)

Remark a: This recommendation applies both to new patients treated with regimens containing 6 months of rifampicin, and to patients returning after default or relapse and now receiving the 8-month retreatment regimen (2HRZES/1HRZE/5HRE). Note that the end of the intensive phase may be at 2 months or 3 months, depending on the regimen.

Remark b: Available evidence showed that smear status at the end of the intensive phase is a poor predictor of relapse, failure and pretreatment isoniazid resistance. Nonetheless, WHO continues to recommend performing smear microscopy at this stage because a positive smear should trigger an assessment of the patient, as well as additional sputum monitoring (see Recommendations 5.2 and 5.3). Sputum smear conversion at the end of the intensive phase is also an indicator of TB programme performance.

■ **Recommendation 5.2**

In new patients, if the specimen obtained at the end of the intensive phase (month 2) is smear-positive, sputum smear microscopy should be obtained at the end of the third month

(Strong/High grade of evidence)

■ **Recommendation 5.3**

In new patients, if the specimen obtained at the end of month 3 is smear-positive, sputum culture and drug susceptibility testing (DST) should be performed

(Strong/High grade of evidence)

Remark: National TB control programmes (NTPs) should continue to follow the current WHO recommendation to obtain sputum specimens for smear microscopy at the end of months 5 and 6 for all new pulmonary TB patients who were smear-positive at the start of treatment. Patients whose sputum smears are positive at month 5 or 6 (or who are found to harbour MDR-TB strains at any time) will be re-registered as having failed treatment and be treated according to Recommendation 7 below.

■ **Recommendation 5.4**

In previously treated patients, if the specimen obtained at the end of the intensive phase (month 3) is smear-positive, sputum culture and drug susceptibility testing (DST) should be performed

(Strong/High grade of evidence)

Question 6. Treatment extension in new pulmonary TB patients

In new pulmonary TB patients, how effective is extension of treatment for preventing failure or relapse?

■ **Recommendation 6**

In patients treated with the regimen containing rifampicin throughout treatment, if a positive sputum smear is found at completion of the intensive phase, the extension of the intensive phase is not recommended

(Strong/High grade of evidence)

Remark: WHO recommends that a positive sputum smear at completion of the intensive phase should trigger a careful review of the quality of patient support and supervision, with prompt intervention if needed (see Chapter 4). It should also trigger additional sputum monitoring, as per Recommendations 5.2, 5.3 and 5.4.

Question 7. Previously treated patients

Which (if any) groups of patients should receive a retreatment regimen with first-line drugs?

Table 3.5 in Chapter 3 shows Recommendations 7.1–7.4.

■ **Recommendation 7.1**

Specimens for culture and drug susceptibility testing (DST) should be obtained from all previously treated TB patients at or before the start of treatment. DST should be performed for at least isoniazid and rifampicin

Remark a: DST may be carried out by rapid molecular-based methods or by conventional methods. Sputum should be obtained, as well as appropriate specimens for extrapulmonary TB, depending on the site of disease.

Remark b: Obtaining specimens for culture and DST should not delay the start of treatment. Empirical therapy should be started promptly, especially if the patient is seriously ill or the disease is progressing rapidly.

■ **Recommendation 7.2**

In settings where rapid molecular-based DST is available, the results should guide the choice of regimen

■ **Recommendation 7.3**

In settings where rapid molecular-based DST results are not routinely available to guide the management of individual patients, empirical[1] treatment should be started as follows:

◾ **Recommendation 7.3.1**

TB patients whose treatment has *failed*[2] or other patient groups with high likelihood of multidrug-resistant TB (MDR-TB) should be started on an empirical MDR regimen

Remark a: In the absence of culture and DST results, the patient should be clinically evaluated before the MDR regimen is administered.

Remark b: Other examples of patients with high likelihood of MDR-TB are those relapsing or defaulting after their second or subsequent course of treatment. See also section 3.8.2.

◾ **Recommendation 7.3.2**

TB patients returning after defaulting or relapsing from their first treatment course may receive the retreatment regimen containing first-line drugs 2HRZES/1HRZE/5HRE if country-specific data show low or medium levels of MDR in these patients or if such data are unavailable

Remark: When DST results become available, regimens should be adjusted appropriately.

■ **Recommendation 7.4**

In settings where DST results are not yet routinely available to guide the management of individual patients, the empirical regimens will continue throughout the course of treatment

■ **Recommendation 7.5**

National TB control programmes should obtain and use their country-specific drug resistance data on failure, relapse and default patient groups to determine the levels of MDR.

---

[1] In these guidelines, empirical means providing treatment before (or without) knowing whether the patient's TB organisms are MDR or not.

[2] Failures in a well-run NTP should be infrequent in the absence of MDR-TB. If they do occur, they are due either to MDR-TB or to programme factors such as poor DOT or poor drug quality. If drug resistance data from failure patients are available and show low or medium levels of MDR, patients should receive the retreatment regimen outlined in section 7.3.2., and every effort should be made to address the underlying programmatic issues.

Remark: Country-specific drug resistance data should include data stratified by type of regimen given for the patient's first course of TB treatment (i.e. 2 vs 6 months of rifampicin).

Table B below lists key changes in this fourth edition, compared to the 2004 update of the third edition.[1]

Table B   KEY CHANGES SINCE THE THIRD EDITION

CHAPTER 1. INTRODUCTION

- The scope is now limited to treatment of TB in adults. The fourth edition no longer covers:
  - TB case detection and diagnosis;
  - diagnosis and treatment of TB in children (WHO has published a separate guideline on management of childhood TB);
  - drug supply management.

- Instead of "Diagnostic categories I–IV", this edition uses the same patient registration groups used for recording and reporting, which differentiate new patients from those with prior treatment and specify reasons for retreatment.

- Each applicable standard from the International Standards for TB Care is cross-referenced.

- An expiry date is provided.

CHAPTER 2. CASE DEFINITIONS

- The recent WHO case definition for sputum smear-positive pulmonary TB[2] has been applied to a definite case of TB, so that now a patient with *one* positive AFB smear is considered a definite case in countries with a functional external quality assurance (EQA) system. (In the third edition, two positive smears were required before a patient could be considered a definite case.)

- Bacteriology now includes culture and new methods for identification of *M. tuberculosis*.

- New WHO data elements for recording and reporting, such as HIV status and MDR-TB, are included.

- Severity of disease is no longer included as a feature of the case definition.

- In the definition for smear-negative TB, this edition incorporates WHO policy reducing the number of specimens from three to two for screening patients suspected to have TB. This policy applies only in settings where a well-functioning EQA system exists, the workload is very high, and human resources are limited.[3]

---

[1] http://www.who.int/tb/publications/cds_tb_2003_313/en/index.html
[2] http://www.who.int/tb/dots/laboratory/policy/en/index1.html
[3] http://www.who.int/tb/dots/laboratory/policy/en/index2.html

- In settings with an HIV prevalence >1% in pregnant women or ≥5% in TB patients, sputum culture for *Mycobacterium tuberculosis* should be performed in patients who are sputum smear-negative to confirm the diagnosis of TB.

- A trial of broad-spectrum antibiotics is no longer recommended to be used as a diagnostic aid for smear-negative pulmonary TB in persons living with HIV.

- For HIV-negative patients, the fourth edition specifies that, if broad-spectrum antibiotics are used in the diagnosis of smear-negative pulmonary TB, anti-TB drugs and fluoroquinolones should be avoided.

- Pulmonary TB cases without smear results are no longer classified as smear-negative. Instead, they are labelled "smear not done" on the TB register and in the annual WHO survey of countries.

- Consistent with Standard 3 of the International Standards for TB Care, culture and histopathological examination are recommended for specimens from suspected extrapulmonary sites of TB. Examination of sputum and a chest radiograph are also suggested, in case patients have concomitant pulmonary involvement.

- The patient registration group "Other" no longer includes "chronic". Instead, patients whose sputum is smear-positive at the end of (or returning from) a second or subsequent course of treatment are classified by the outcome of their most recent retreatment course: relapsed, defaulted or failed.

CHAPTER 3. STANDARD TREATMENT REGIMENS

- Additional dosage information is provided for isoniazid (maximum daily dose for three times per week) and streptomycin (maximum dose, and adjustments in persons aged over 60 years or weighing less than 50 kg). Thioacetazone is no longer included among the first-line drugs.

- A new section on TB patient kits has been added.

- The recommended new patient regimen contains 6 months of rifampicin; the regimen with 2 months of rifampicin (with the 6-month continuation phase of isoniazid and ethambutol) is no longer an option.

- In this edition, three times weekly dosing throughout therapy is an alternative only for patients who are receiving directly observed therapy of every dose and who are not HIV-positive or living in an HIV-prevalent setting. Three times weekly dosing during the intensive phase is no longer an option for HIV-positive TB patients or TB patients living in HIV-prevalent settings.

- WHO now recommends against twice weekly dosing for the full course of treatment for new patients (unless done in the context of formal research).The third edition included the option to omit ethambutol during the intensive phase of treatment for patients with non-cavitary, smear-negative pulmonary TB or extrapulmonary disease who are known to be HIV-negative. In the fourth edition, the omission of ethambutol is no longer recommended.

- This fourth edition includes an alternative continuation phase of ethambutol, rifampicin, and isoniazid for new patients in populations with high levels of isoniazid resistance. This conditional recommendation applies where isoniazid susceptibility testing in new patients is not done (or results are not available) before the continuation phase begins.

- DST before or at the start of therapy is strongly recommended for all previously treated patients.

- Previously treated patients are defined by their likelihood of MDR-TB, and recommendations for treatment regimen depend on reason for retreatment (failure, versus relapse and default).

- Laboratory tests (liquid media, line probe assays) to meet the needs for the prompt identification of *M. tuberculosis* and DST are discussed, based on country-specific, comprehensive plans for laboratory strengthening.

- Guidance for starting therapy is provided for previously treated patients, based on whether the country has access to new rapid molecular-based tests, access to conventional DST, or no routine access to DST results to guide management of individual patients.

- In countries using conventional DST, a standard empirical MDR regimen is recommended for patients with high likelihood of MDR, while awaiting DST results. When DST results become available, regimens should be adjusted appropriately.

- An MDR regimen is now recommended as one of each country's standard regimens, for use in confirmed MDR-TB cases as well as in patients with a high likelihood of MDR while awaiting DST results. This edition also gives interim guidance to countries where DST is not yet routinely available for individual retreatment patients.

- Given the availability of funding from international financial mechanisms, lack of resources for MDR treatment is no longer an acceptable rationale for providing a retreatment regimen of first-line drugs (formerly called the "Category 2 regimen") to patients with a high likelihood of MDR.

- The previous edition recommended the 8-month retreatment regimen with first-line drugs for all TB patients returning after defaulting or relapsing. By contrast, this edition allows for the possibility that, in some countries, these patients may have levels of MDR-TB that are high enough to warrant an MDR regimen while awaiting results of DST.

- WHO does not intend to establish thresholds for low, moderate, or high likelihoods or levels of MDR. NTPs will define "low," "moderate" and "high" for their own countries, based on levels of MDR in specific patient groups, as well as other factors such as MDR treatment resources available during scale-up, and frequency of concomitant conditions (such as HIV) that increase the short-term risk of dying from MDR-TB.

- Country drug resistance surveys, WHO estimates of MDR levels, and other data sources are recommended to inform decisions on each country's standard treatment regimens for defined patient groups.

- Intermittent dosing is no longer an option for previously treated patients receiving the 8-month retreatment regimen with first-line drugs.

CHAPTER 4. MONITORING DURING TREATMENT

- The performance of sputum smear microscopy at the completion of the intensive phase of treatment is a conditional, rather than a strong, recommendation, given the evidence that a positive smear at this stage has a very poor ability to predict relapse or pretreatment isoniazid resistance (Annex 2). However, its utility in detecting problems with patient supervision and for monitoring programme performance is reaffirmed.

- In addition, this edition recommends that a positive sputum smear at the end of the intensive phase in new patients should trigger sputum smear microscopy at the end of the third month. If the latter is positive, culture and DST should be performed.

- This edition no longer recommends extension of the intensive phase for patients who have a positive sputum smear at the end of the second month of treatment.

- In previously treated patients, if the specimen obtained at the end of the intensive phase (month 3) is smear-positive, this edition recommends that sputum culture and DST be performed then, rather than waiting until month 5 (which was recommended in the third edition).

- The outcome of cure now encompasses culture results.

- Patients found to harbour an MDR-TB strain at any point during treatment are now classified as "treatment failure". They are re-registered and begin an MDR regimen.

- For MDR-TB patients, this edition recommends the use of the MDR-TB register and cohort analysis.

- The symptom-based approach to side-effects of anti-TB drugs has been revised.

CHAPTER 5. CO-MANAGEMENT OF HIV AND ACTIVE TB DISEASE

- Provider-initiated HIV testing for all patients with known or suspected TB is now recommended, regardless of the stage of the country's HIV epidemic.

- This edition includes current WHO recommendations to start co-trimoxazole as soon as possible when a person living with HIV is diagnosed with TB.

- Daily dosing is strongly recommended during the intensive phase for TB patients with known positive HIV status, and all new patients living in HIV-prevalent settings. Three times per week dosing during the intensive phase is no longer an acceptable alternative.

- Current WHO recommendations for antiretroviral therapy and timing of initiation are incorporated.

- Drug susceptibility testing is now recommended at the start of TB therapy in all people living with HIV.

CHAPTER 6. SUPERVISION AND PATIENT SUPPORT

- Roles of the patient, TB programme staff, the community, and other providers are described in assuring adherence to treatment. A treatment supporter must be identified for each TB patient, which may be a health worker, or a trained and supervised member of the community or family.

- Treatment supervision is defined in the context of a larger support package to address patients' needs.

CHAPTER 7. TREATMENT OF DRUG-RESISTANT TB

- This chapter has been extensively revised to reflect recent WHO recommendations for the programmatic management of drug-resistant TB.

CHAPTER 8. TB TREATMENT OF EXTRAPULMONARY DISEASE AND OF TB IN SPECIAL SITUATIONS

- While WHO continues to recommend the same regimens for extrapulmonary and pulmonary disease, this fourth edition references other guidelines suggesting longer treatment for TB meningitis and for bone or joint TB.

- For TB patients with pre-existing liver disease, this fourth edition includes regimens with one, two and no hepatotoxic drugs. A 9-month regimen of rifampicin and ethambutol is no longer included as an option.

- For TB patients with renal failure, this edition recommends the 6-month regimen with isoniazid, rifampicin, ethambutol and pyrazinamide, whereas the prior edition omitted pyrazinamide. This edition recommends administering ethambutol (15 mg/kg) and pyrazinamide (25 mg/kg) three times per week. This edition now discourages the use of streptomycin in patients with renal failure; however, if it must be used, 15 mg/kg should be administered two to three times per week, with monitoring of drug levels.

Annex 1

- Rifampicin: includes a list of drugs which interact with rifampicin.

- Streptomycin: dosage adjustments for the elderly and adults weighing less than 50 kg are provided.

- Ethambutol: creatinine clearance <50 ml/min is no longer listed as a contraindication. Dosage adjustment in renal failure is provided.

Annex 2

- This new annex describes the evidence base and issues that were considered in making recommendations.

Annex 3

- This annex describes the most critical treatment outcomes considered.

Annex 4

- In this new annex, steps for implementing and evaluating the strong recommendations are described.

Annex 5

- This annex provides suggestions for future research under each of the seven questions.

Annex 6

- This new annex lists the members of the Guidelines Group and the External Review Group.

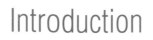

Introduction

1.1 Chapter objectives

This chapter defines the purpose, target audience, scope and development of this fourth edition of the guidelines. It also explains why a new edition was needed and projects a date for the next revision.

1.2 Purpose of the guidelines

The principal purpose of these guidelines is to help national TB control programmes (NTPs) in setting TB treatment policy to optimize patient cure: curing patients will prevent death, relapse, acquired drug resistance, and the spread of TB in the community. Their further purpose is to guide clinicians working in both public and private sectors.

1.3 Target audience

The primary target audience for the guidelines is the managers and staff of NTPs, together with other TB service providers working in public and private health care facilities at the central and peripheral levels.

Use of the term "NTP manager" in these guidelines refers to the official within, or designated by, the ministry of health who is responsible for the TB programme or to that official's designee.

1.4 Scope

These guidelines address the treatment of active TB disease in adults. They exclude many related topics that have already been covered in detail in other publications: diagnosis, laboratory standards for smear microscopy, protocols for use of rapid drug susceptibility tests, paediatric TB, drug procurement and supply management, infection control, intensified case-finding in persons living with HIV, and isoniazid preventive therapy.

1.5 Why a new edition?

Major progress in global TB control followed the widespread implementation of the DOTS strategy. The Stop TB Strategy, launched in 2006, builds upon and enhances the achievements of DOTS (1): new objectives include universal access to patient-centred treatment, and protection of populations from TB/HIV coinfection and multidrug-resistant TB (MDR-TB). The Stop TB Strategy and the Global Plan (2) to implement the new strategy made it necessary to revise the existing guidelines (3) and develop this fourth edition.

Historically, the greatest emphasis of TB control activities has been on the most infectious patients – those who have sputum smear-positive pulmonary tuberculosis (3). This changed with the Stop TB Strategy's emphasis on universal access for all persons with TB to high-quality, patient-centred treatment (1). However, highly infectious, smear-positive patients remain the primary focus for other aspects of TB control, including contact tracing and infection control. The Patients' Charter for TB Care specifies that all TB patients have "the right to free and equitable access to TB care, from diagnosis through treatment completion" (4).

This fourth edition of the guidelines has therefore abandoned Categories I–IV, which were used to prioritize patients for treatment.[1] According to this prior categorization, smear-negative TB patients were assigned third priority and MDR-TB patients fourth priority. For treatment decisions it no longer makes sense to assign third priority to smear-negative patients given their high mortality if they are living with HIV. Equally, MDR-TB patients should not be assigned fourth priority, given their high mortality and the urgent need to prevent the spread of these deadliest TB strains.

To replace Categories I–IV, this fourth edition groups patients (and standard regimens recommended for each group) according to the likelihood of their having drug resistance. Drug resistance is a critical determinant of treatment success, and prior TB treatment confers an increased risk (5, 6). This edition uses the same patient registration groups as those used for recording and reporting, which differentiate new patients from those who have had prior treatment (7). Registration groups for previously treated patients are based on the outcome of their prior treatment course: failure, relapse, and default.

The fourth edition integrates detection and treatment of both HIV infection and MDR-TB, and thus should contribute towards achievement of the Stop TB Strategy's universal access to high-quality MDR-TB and HIV care.

With regard to HIV detection, this edition incorporates recent WHO recommendations for provider-initiated HIV testing of all persons with diagnosed or suspected TB, in all types of HIV epidemics (low-level, concentrated or generalized) (8). For treatment of TB in persons living with HIV, new recommendations on the duration of therapy and the role of intermittent regimens have emerged from systematic reviews (see Chapter 5). The new edition also includes recent WHO recommendations for DST at the start of TB therapy in all people living with HIV (9), as well as recommendations on the timing and type of antiretroviral therapy (ART) regimens (10).

---

[1] Also, the original one-to-one correspondence between patient group and treatment regimens was lost as Categories I–IV were redefined over the years. The same treatment regimen came to be recommended for patients in Categories I and III; after 2004, different treatment regimens were recommended for patients in Category II depending on factors such as programme performance and drug resistance.

New developments in MDR-TB also contributed to the need for this revision. Building on the principle of universal access to MDR-TB diagnosis and care, *The MDR-TB and XDR-TB response plan 2007–2008* (*11*) calls for the diagnosis and treatment of MDR-TB in all countries by 2015. Even countries with low overall levels of multidrug resistance (MDR) are faced with TB patients who have been previously treated – a group that is five times more likely to have MDR-TB than new patients (see section 3.6).

In terms of ensuring universal access to MDR-TB diagnosis, this fourth edition reaffirms existing WHO recommendations (*2*) that all previously treated patients should have access to culture and DST at the beginning of treatment, in order to identify MDR-TB as early as possible.[1] It also incorporates the WHO recommendation that treatment failure be confirmed by culture and DST (*9*). In order to detect MDR sooner than the end of the fifth month of treatment, this edition includes the existing WHO recommendation (*9*) for culture and DST if patients still have smear-positive sputum at the end of the third month of treatment.

Chapters 2–5 of this new edition discuss the critical role of the identification of *Mycobacterium tuberculosis* and of DST. This is in contrast to the previous edition, which relied almost exclusively on smear microscopy for case definition, assignment of standard regimens, and monitoring of treatment response. Line probe assays can identify MDR-TB within hours and liquid media can do so within weeks (rather than months when solid media are used) (*12*). These techniques should be introduced in line with comprehensive, country-specific plans for laboratory capacity strengthening.

To move towards universal access to MDR-TB treatment, the fourth edition includes a new recommendation for every country to include an MDR regimen in its standard regimens. This is essential while awaiting DST results for patients with a high likelihood of MDR (such as those whose prior treatment with a 6-month rifampicin regimen has failed), and for patients in whom resistance to isoniazid and rifampicin is confirmed. With the availability of funding from international financial partners,[2] lack of resources for MDR-TB treatment is no longer an acceptable rationale for providing the 8-month retreatment regimen with first-line drugs (formerly called the "Category II regimen") to patients with a high likelihood of MDR; this regimen is ineffective in treating MDR-TB and may result in amplification of drug resistance (*5, 13*).

Use of rapid DST methods will eventually render the 8-month retreatment regimen of first-line drugs obsolete. In the meantime, the regimen is retained in this fourth edition in only two circumstances. In countries with access to routine DST using conventional methods, the 8-month retreatment regimen with first-line drugs is recommended while awaiting DST results from patients who have relapsed or are returning after default (if country-specific data show they have a medium likelihood

---

[1] This recommendation is consistent with the International Standards for Tuberculosis Care and resolutions endorsed by the World Health Assembly in 2007 which call for universal access to DST by 2015.
[2] Such as UNITAID and the Global Fund to Fight AIDS, Tuberculosis and Malaria.

of MDR-TB, or if such data are unavailable). In countries that do not yet have DST routinely available at the start of treatment for all previously treated patients (see section 3.7.3), the 8-month retreatment regimen with first-line drugs will be used for the duration of treatment on an interim basis until laboratory capacity is available.

In principle, MDR treatment should be introduced only in well-performing DOTS programmes. Before focusing on curing MDR-TB cases, it is critical to "turn off the tap", i.e. to strengthen poor programmes so that they stop giving rise to MDR-TB. Following this principle, the 2004 revision of the treatment chapter[1] listed adequate performance of a country's overall TB programme as a requirement for the use of MDR regimens in patients with a high likelihood of MDR. This is no longer a prerequisite in the fourth edition. In some countries with limited DOTS coverage, there may be an appropriate setting for an MDR pilot project that, once established, can provide a model and an impetus for the expansion of basic DOTS into more areas. In most countries, however, conditions for initiating an MDR component in most NTPs are not met until the overall NTP has the essential elements of DOTS firmly in place.

1.6 Methodology

Development of the fourth edition of the guidelines followed new WHO procedures. WHO defined the scope of revision and convened a guidelines group of external experts. All members of the group completed a Declaration for the Conflict of Interest; there were no conflicts declared. With input from the Guidelines Group, WHO identified seven key questions on the treatment of TB (see Annex 2) covering the following topics:

— duration of rifampicin in new patients;
— dosing frequency in new patients;
— initial regimen for new TB patients in countries with high levels of isoniazid resistance;
— TB treatment in persons living with HIV;
— sputum monitoring during TB treatment;
— treatment extension;
— retreatment.

Systematic literature reviews were conducted for each question and the evidence was synthesized[2] (see Annex 2).

Input from the Guidelines Group to the revision of guidelines was made by e-mail, in conference calls and at a 3-day meeting (21–23 October 2008) during which the final treatment recommendations were established once consensus had been reached by

---

[1] *Treatment of tuberculosis: guidelines for national programmes*, 3rd ed. Chapter 4, Standard treatment regimens, was revised in June 2004 and the new version was posted on the WHO web site.
[2] At the time of publication of this fourth edition, evidence gathered through some of the systematic reviews had not been published.

the Guidelines Group. The recommendations are based on the quality of the evidence, values, and costs, as well as judgements about trade-offs between benefits and harm.

The group graded the strength of each recommendation, reflecting the degree of confidence that the desirable effects of adherence to a recommendation outweigh the undesirable effects. Although the degree of confidence is necessarily a continuum, three categories are used – strong, conditional and weak. The quality of the evidence was assessed according to the GRADE methodology (14).

Moderate/low quality of evidence means that the estimate of effect of the intervention is very uncertain and further research is likely to have an important impact on confidence in the estimate. For high-quality evidence, by contrast, further research is unlikely to change confidence in the estimate of effect.

A strong recommendation means that the desirable effects of adherence to the recommendation clearly outweigh the undesirable effects. Strong recommendations use the words "should" or "should not". No alternatives are listed.

A conditional recommendation means that the desirable effects of adherence to the recommendation probably outweigh the undesirable effects, but the trade-offs are uncertain. Reasons for lack of certainty include:

— high-quality evidence to support the recommendation is lacking;
— benefits of implementing the recommendation are small;
— benefits may not justify the costs;
— it was not possible to arrive at precise estimates of benefit.

A weak recommendation means that there is insufficient evidence; the recommendation is therefore based on field application and expert opinion.

Conditional and weak recommendations use the word "may". Alternatives are listed for several of the conditional recommendations.

Table 1.1 shows how strong and conditional recommendations differ in terms both of wording and of the factors used to judge their strength. Strong and conditional recommendations also have different implications for policy-makers, patients, and health care providers; these are summarized in the table.

A plan for implementing and evaluating the strong recommendations is outlined in Annex 4. To address the gaps in the evidence critical for decision-making, the Guidelines Group developed a series of questions as a basis for future research; these are detailed in Annex 5. Members of the Guidelines Group are listed in Annex 6.

The recommendations that address the seven key questions appear in the context of guidance on standard treatment (Chapter 3), monitoring (Chapter 4) and HIV (Chapter 5). Areas outside the scope of those questions have been updated with current references and WHO TB policies but were not the subject of systematic literature reviews or of new recommendations by the Guidelines Group.

Table 1.1   STRONG VERSUS CONDITIONAL RECOMMENDATIONS

	Recommendation strength	
	Strong	**Conditional**
Phrasing of the recommendation	**"Should"** or **"should not"**. No alternatives are presented	**"Optimal is"**, **"may"**, or **"it is (not) recommended"**. Alternatives are often listed
Factors used to judge strength		
Quality of evidence	High-quality evidence	Low-quality evidence
Balance between desirable and undesirable effects on patient and public health	Large, certain net benefit and/or difference between benefits and harms or burdens	Small and/or uncertain gradient
Resource allocation	Low cost (or little uncertainty about whether the intervention represents a wise use of resources)	High cost (or high uncertainty)
Uncertainty in values and preferences; variability across patients	Small amount of uncertainty or variability	Large amount of uncertainty or variability
Implications		
For policy-makers (including NTP managers)	The recommendation should unequivocally be used for setting policy	Policy-making will require extensive debate
For patients	Most individuals would want the recommended course of action	The recommended course of action can be adjusted on the basis of feasibility and acceptability
For health care providers	Most patients should be treated according to the recommended course of action. Adherence to this recommendation is a reasonable measure of good quality care	

The draft guidelines were circulated to the external review group (whose members are listed in Annex 6), made up of NTP managers from high-burden countries, members of the WHO Strategic, Technical and Advisory Group on TB (STAG-TB), six regional TB Advisers and TB medical officers working in high-burden countries.

Comments received from the external review group were appropriately addressed and the few disagreements between the external reviewers and the Guidelines Group were resolved by e-mail consultation.

1.7 International Standards for Tuberculosis Care

The *International Standards for Tuberculosis Care* (ISTC) (*15*) describe a widely accepted level of TB care that all practitioners should seek to achieve. Cross-referencing the applicable ISTC standards in this new edition should help providers in both public and private sectors to ensure their implementation.

1.8 Expiry date

The WHO Stop TB Department will review and update these guidelines after 3–5 years or as needed when new evidence, treatment regimens or diagnostic tests become available.

References

1. Raviglione MC, Uplekar MW. WHO's new stop TB strategy. *Lancet,* 2006, 367:952–955.
2. *The global plan to stop TB, 2006–2015.* Geneva, World Health Organization, 2006 (WHO/HTM/STB/2006.35).
3. *Treatment of tuberculosis: guidelines for national programmes*, 3rd ed. Geneva, World Health Organization, 2003 (WHO/CDS/TB/2003.313).
4. *Patients' charter for tuberculosis care: patients' rights and responsibilities.* Geneva, World Care Council, 2006 (available at: www.who.int/tb/publications/2006/patients_charter.pdf).
5. Espinal MA et al. Standard short-course chemotherapy for drug-resistant tuberculosis: treatment outcomes in 6 countries. *Journal of the American Medical Association,* 2000, 283:2537–2545.
6. Aziz MA et al. Epidemiology of antituberculosis drug resistance (the Global Project on Anti-tuberculosis Drug Resistance Surveillance): an updated analysis. *Lancet,* 2006, 368:2142–2154.
7. *Revised TB recording and reporting forms and registers – version 2006.* Geneva, World Health Organization, 2006 (WHO/HTM/TB/2006.373; available at: www.who.int/tb/dots/r_and_r_forms/en/index.html).
8. *Guidance on provider-initiated HIV testing and counselling in health facilities.* Geneva, World Health Organization, 2007.
9. *Guidelines for the programmatic management of drug-resistant tuberculosis: emergency update 2008.* Geneva, World Health Organization, 2008 (WHO/HTM/TB/2008.402).

10. *Antiretroviral therapy for HIV infection in adults and adolescents in resource-limited settings: recommendations for a public health approach*. Geneva, World Health Organization, 2006.

11. *The global MDR-TB & XDR-TB response plan 2007–2008*. Geneva, World Health Organization, 2007 (WHO/HTM/TB/2007.387).

12. *Molecular line probe assays for rapid screening of patients at risk of MDR TB: policy statement*. Geneva, World Health Organization, 2008 (available at: www.who.int/tb/features_archive/policy_statement.pdf).

13. Espinal MA. Time to abandon the standard retreatment regimen with first-line drugs for failures of standard treatment. *International Journal of Tuberculosis and Lung Disease*, 2003, 7:607–608.

14. Guyatt GH et al. GRADE: an emerging consensus on rating quality of evidence and strength of recommendations. *British Medical Journal*, 2008, 336:924–926.

15. *International Standards for Tuberculosis Care (ISTC)*, 2nd ed. The Hague, Tuberculosis Coalition for Technical Assistance, 2009.

Case definitions

2.1 Chapter objectives

This chapter describes

— the purpose of having case definitions for tuberculosis;
— the definition of a case of TB, as well as of suspected and confirmed cases;
— additional features of TB cases important for the treatment of individual patients, as well as for evaluating TB programmes and monitoring the epidemic.

The diagnosis of TB refers to the recognition by health workers (medical officer, nurse, paramedic or other) of an active case, i.e. a patient with current disease due to *M. tuberculosis*. The role of NTPs is different: they are responsible for ensuring that diagnosed cases are notified (*1*), meet the definition for case or definite case, and are treated appropriately, and that outcomes are evaluated.[1]

All providers must report both new and retreatment TB cases and their treatment outcomes to local public health authorities, in conformance with applicable legal requirements (Standard 21 of the ISTC (*5*)). NTPs ensure that critical features of the TB case are recorded and reported so that treatment is appropriate and feedback is provided to the treating clinician (*6*). Analysis of these reports also helps the NTP manager to monitor trends and evaluate the effectiveness of TB activities at all levels.

2.2 Purposes of defining a TB case

Uniform criteria to define a TB case are needed for:

— proper patient registration and case notification;
— selecting appropriate standard treatment regimens (see Chapter 3);
— standardizing the process of data collection for TB control;
— evaluating the proportion of cases according to site, bacteriology and treatment history;
— cohort analysis of treatment outcomes;
— accurate monitoring of trends and evaluation of the effectiveness of TB programmes within and across districts, countries and global regions.

2.3 Case definitions

The TB case definitions below are based on the level of certainty of the diagnosis and on whether or not laboratory confirmation is available.

---

[1] NTP programmes also facilitate the detection of cases via sputum screening of suspects with cough attending health facilities (*2*), as well as screening of contacts (*3*) and screening of persons living with HIV/AIDS (*4*).

- **Tuberculosis suspect**. Any person who presents with symptoms or signs suggestive of TB. The most common symptom of pulmonary TB is a productive cough for more than 2 weeks,[1] which may be accompanied by other respiratory symptoms (shortness of breath, chest pains, haemoptysis) and/or constitutional symptoms (loss of appetite, weight loss, fever, night sweats, and fatigue).[2]

- **Case of tuberculosis**. A definite case of TB (defined below) or one in which a health worker (clinician or other medical practitioner) has diagnosed TB and has decided to treat the patient with a full course of TB treatment.

  Note. Any person given treatment for TB should be recorded as a case. Incomplete "trial" TB treatment should not be given as a method for diagnosis.

- **Definite case of tuberculosis**. A patient with *Mycobacterium tuberculosis* complex identified from a clinical specimen, either by culture or by a newer method such as molecular line probe assay. In countries that lack the laboratory capacity to routinely identify *M. tuberculosis*, a pulmonary case with one or more initial sputum smear examinations positive for acid-fast bacilli (AFB) is also considered to be a "definite" case, provided that there is a functional external quality assurance (EQA) system with blind rechecking.[3]

Cases of TB are also classified according to the:

— anatomical site of disease;
— bacteriological results (including drug resistance);
— history of previous treatment;
— HIV status of the patient.

Each of these key features of TB cases is discussed below.

2.4 Anatomical site of TB disease

In general, recommended treatment regimens are similar, irrespective of site (see section 8.2). Defining the site is important for recording and reporting purposes and to identify the more infectious patients – those with pulmonary involvement (who will be further subdivided by smear status – see section 2.5 below).

Pulmonary tuberculosis (PTB) refers to a case of TB (defined above) involving the lung parenchyma. Miliary tuberculosis is classified as pulmonary TB because there are lesions in the lungs. Tuberculous intrathoracic lymphadenopathy (mediastinal and/or hilar) or tuberculous pleural effusion, without radiographic abnormalities in the lungs, constitutes a case of *extra*pulmonary TB. A patient with both pulmonary and extrapulmonary TB should be classified as a case of *pulmonary* TB.

---

[1] Standard 1 of the International Standards for TB Care (5) states that all persons with otherwise unexplained productive cough lasting 2–3 weeks or more should be evaluated for TB.
[2] The definition of a "TB suspect" depends on other local factors, including the patient's age and HIV status, HIV prevalence in the population, TB prevalence in the population, etc.
[3] See: www.who.int/tb/dots/laboratory/policy/en/index1.html.

Extrapulmonary tuberculosis (EPTB) refers to a case of TB (defined above) involving organs other than the lungs, e.g. pleura, lymph nodes, abdomen, genitourinary tract, skin, joints and bones, meninges. Diagnosis should be based on at least one specimen with confirmed *M. tuberculosis* or histological or strong clinical evidence consistent with active EPTB, followed by a decision by a clinician to treat with a full course of tuberculosis chemotherapy. The case definition of an EPTB case with several sites affected depends on the site representing the most severe form of disease. Unless a case of EPTB is confirmed by culture as caused by *M. tuberculosis*, it cannot meet the "definite case" definition given in section 2.3 above.

2.5 Bacteriological results

Bacteriology refers to the smear status of pulmonary cases and the identification of *M. tuberculosis* for any case by culture or newer methods. Culture and drug susceptibility testing are discussed in section 3.8.1. For definitions of MDR-TB cases, see reference 7.

Standard 2 of the ISTC (5) states that all patients suspected of having pulmonary TB should submit at least two sputum specimens for microscopic examination in a quality-assured laboratory. When possible, at least one early-morning specimen should be obtained, as sputum collected at this time has the highest yield. ISTC Standard 4 states that all persons with chest radiographic findings suggestive of TB should submit sputum specimens for microbiological examination (5).

Smear-positive cases are the most infectious and most likely to transmit their disease in their surroundings; they are the focus for infection control measures (2) and contact investigations (3). Bacteriological monitoring of treatment progress is most feasible and practicable in these patients (see Chapter 4).

It is also important to identify smear-negative cases, especially in persons living with HIV for whom mortality is higher than in smear-positive pulmonary TB cases (4). For diagnostic algorithms for smear-negative persons living with HIV, see reference 4.

A case of pulmonary TB is considered to be *smear-positive* if one or more sputum smear specimens at the start of treatment are positive for AFB (provided that there is a functional EQA system with blind rechecking[1]).

The definition of a new sputum smear-positive pulmonary TB case is based on the presence of at least one acid fast bacillus (AFB+) in at least one sputum sample in countries with a well functioning EQA system. (See www.who.int/tb/dots/laboratory/policy/en/index1.html.)

---

[1] In countries without functional EQA, the definition from the third edition of these guidelines applies: a smear-positive pulmonary TB case was defined as one with:

a. two or more initial sputum smear examinations positive for AFB, **or**

b. one sputum smear examination positive for AFB plus radiographic abnormalities consistent with active PTB as determined by a clinician, **or**

c. one sputum smear positive for AFB plus sputum culture-positive for *M. tuberculosis*.

Smear-negative PTB cases should either:

A. have sputum that is smear-negative but culture-positive for *M. tuberculosis*:

- a case of pulmonary TB is considered to be *smear-negative* if at least two sputum specimens at the start of treatment are negative for AFB[1] in countries with a functional EQA system, where the workload is very high and human resources are limited (see http:///www.who.int/tb/dots/laboratory/policy/en/index2.html);

- in all settings with an HIV prevalence of >1% in pregnant women or ≥5% in TB patients, sputum culture for *M. tuberculosis* should be performed in patients who are sputum smear-negative to confirm the diagnosis of TB (4).

OR

B. meet the following diagnostic criteria: (6–8)

- decision by a clinician to treat with a full course of anti-TB therapy; and

- radiographic abnormalities consistent with active pulmonary TB and *either*:
  — laboratory or strong clinical evidence of HIV infection

  or:

  — if HIV-negative (or unknown HIV status living in an area of low HIV prevalence), no improvement in response to a course of broad-spectrum antibiotics (excluding anti-TB drugs and fluoroquinolones and aminoglycosides).

Pulmonary TB cases without smear results are no longer classified as smear-negative (4); instead, they are recorded as "smear not done" on the TB register (6) and on the annual WHO survey of countries.

For patients suspected of having EPTB, specimens should be obtained from the suspected sites of involvement (Standard 3 of the ISTC (5)). Where available, culture and histopathological examination should also be carried out. Additionally, a chest X-ray and examination of sputum may be useful, especially in persons with HIV infection.

2.6 History of previous treatment: patient registration group

At the time of registration, each patient meeting the case definition is also classified according to whether or not he or she has previously received TB treatment and, if so, the outcome (if known). It is important to identify previously treated patients because they are at increased risk of drug resistance, including MDR-TB (see section 3.6). At the start of therapy, specimens should be obtained for culture and DST from all previously treated patients. Treatment depends on whether the patient has relapsed

---

[1] And no specimen is smear-positive.

or is returning after default or after prior treatment has failed (see section 3.7). The distinctions between new and previously treated patients, and among the subgroups of previously treated patients, are also essential for monitoring the TB epidemic and programme performance.

New patients have never had treatment for TB, or have taken anti-TB drugs for less than 1 month. New patients may have positive or negative bacteriology and may have disease at any anatomical site.

Previously treated patients have received 1 month or more of anti-TB drugs in the past, may have positive or negative bacteriology and may have disease at any anatomical site. They are further classified by the outcome of their most recent course of treatment as shown in Table 2.1 below.

Patients whose sputum is smear-positive at the end of (or returning from) a second or subsequent course of treatment are no longer defined as "chronic". Instead, they should be classified by the outcome of their most recent retreatment course: relapsed, defaulted or failed.

Table 2.1   REGISTRATION GROUP BY OUTCOME OF MOST RECENT TB TREATMENT

Registration group (any site of disease)		Bacteriology[a]	Outcome of most recent prior treatment (defined in Table 4.1)
New		+ or −	−
Previously treated	**Relapse**	+	Cured
			Treatment completed
	Failure	+	Treatment failed
	Default	+	Defaulted
Transfer in: A patient who has been transferred from another TB register to continue treatment		+ or −	Still on treatment
Other		+ or −	All cases that do not fit the above definitions, such as patients <ul><li>for whom it is not known whether they have been previously treated;</li><li>who were previously treated but with unknown outcome of that previous treatment[b] (*3, 8*); and/or</li><li>who have returned to treatment with smear-negative PTB or bacteriologically negative EPTB[b] (*3*)</li></ul>

[a]   + indicates positive smear, culture or other newer means of identifying *M. tuberculosis*
    − indicates that any specimens tested were negative.
[b]   Defined as "other retreatment" in other WHO documents cited above.

2.7 HIV status

Determining and recording the patient's HIV status is critical for treatment decisions (see Chapters 3 and 5) as well as for monitoring trends and assessing programme performance. WHO's revised TB Treatment Card and TB Register include dates of HIV testing, starting co-trimoxazole, and starting ART. These important interventions are discussed more fully in Chapter 5.

References

1. *Engaging all health care providers in TB control: guidance on implementing public-private mix approaches.* Geneva, World Health Organization, 2006 (WHO/HTM/TB/2006.360).

2. *WHO policy on TB infection control in health care facilities, congregate settings and households.* Geneva, World Health Organization, 2009 (WHO/HTM/TB/2009.419).

3. *Implementing the WHO Stop TB Strategy: a handbook for national tuberculosis control programmes.* Geneva, World Health Organization, 2008 (WHO/HTM/TB/2008.40).

4. *Improving the diagnosis and treatment of smear-negative pulmonary and extrapulmonary tuberculosis among adults and adolescents: recommendations for HIV-prevalent and resource-constrained settings.* Geneva, World Health Organization, 2007 (WHO/HTM/TB/2007.379; WHO/HIV/2007.1).

5. *International Standards for Tuberculosis Care (ISTC),* 2nd ed. The Hague, Tuberculosis Coalition for Technical Assistance, 2009.

6. *Revised TB recording and reporting forms and registers – version 2006.* Geneva, World Health Organization, 2006 (WHO/HTM/TB/2006.373; available at: www.who.int/tb/dots/r_and_r_forms/en/index.html).

7. *Guidelines for the programmatic management of drug-resistant tuberculosis: emergency update 2008.* Geneva, World Health Organization, 2008 (WHO/HTM/TB/2008.402).

8. *Global tuberculosis control 2009: epidemiology, strategy, financing. WHO report 2009.* Geneva, World Health Organization, 2009 (WHO/HTM/TB/2009.411).

Standard treatment regimens

3.1 Chapter objectives

This chapter describes:

— the aims of treatment;
— the recommended doses of first-line anti-TB drugs for adults;
— regimens for new and previously treated patients;
— considerations in selecting regimens for defined patient groups;
— evidence base for the selected regimens in defined patient groups.

The choice of TB regimens in special situations (pregnancy, concurrent use of oral contraceptives, liver disease, and renal failure) is covered in Chapter 8; TB treatment for persons living with HIV is discussed in Chapter 5.

3.2 Aims of treatment

The aims of treatment of tuberculosis are:

— to cure the patient and restore quality of life and productivity;
— to prevent death from active TB or its late effects;
— to prevent relapse of TB;
— to reduce transmission of TB to others;
— to prevent the development and transmission of drug resistance.

3.3 Essential antituberculosis drugs

Table 3.1 shows the essential anti-TB drugs and their recommended dosages based on the patient's weight.

The WHO-recommended formulations of anti-TB drugs and fixed-dose combinations (FDCs) of drugs appear in the *WHO Model List of Essential Medicines* (available at www.who.int/medicines/publications/essentialmedicines/en). The formulations and combinations of anti-TB drugs available in each country should conform to this list. (See also the WHO Model Formulary at www.who.int/selection_medicines/list/en.)

To facilitate procurement, distribution and administration of treatment to patients, the daily dosage may be standardized for three or four body weight bands – for instance 30–39 kg, 40–54 kg, 55–70 kg and over 70 kg, as is done with the Global Drug Facility patient kits. (See also reference *1*.)

Table 3.1   RECOMMENDED DOSES OF FIRST-LINE ANTITUBERCULOSIS DRUGS
FOR ADULTS

Drug	Daily Dose and range (mg/kg body weight)	Daily Maximum (mg)	3 times per week Dose and range (mg/kg body weight)	3 times per week Daily maximum (mg)
Isoniazid	5 (4–6)	300	10 (8–12)	900
Rifampicin	10 (8–12)	600	10 (8–12)	600
Pyrazinamide	25 (20–30)	–	35 (30–40)	–
Ethambutol	15 (15–20)	–	30 (25–35)	–
Streptomycin[a]	15 (12–18)		15 (12–18)	1000

[a] Patients aged over 60 years may not be able to tolerate more than 500–750 mg daily, so some guidelines recommend reduction of the dose to 10 mg/kg per day in patients in this age group (*2*). Patients weighing less than 50 kg may not tolerate doses above 500–750 mg daily (*WHO Model Formulary 2008*, www.who.int/selection_medicines/list/en/).

All anti-TB drugs should be quality-assured, and management of anti-TB drugs should be incorporated into the management of other essential medicines by the ministry of health.

Annex 1 provides additional information on the essential anti-TB drugs, including contraindications, precautions, use in pregnancy, adverse effects, and drug interactions. Intermittent dosing schedules are discussed in section 3.5.1 below.

3.3.1   Fixed-dose combinations of anti-TB drugs

While evidence on fixed-dose combinations (FDCs) of anti-TB drugs was not systematically reviewed for this fourth edition, WHO continues to recommend their use, as does Standard 8 of the ISTC (*3*). FDCs are thought to prevent acquisition of drug resistance due to monotherapy, which may occur with separate ("loose") drugs. With FDCs, patients cannot be selective in the choice of drugs to ingest. Prescription errors are likely to be less frequent because dosage recommendations are more straightforward, and adjustment of dosage according to patient weight is easier. The number of tablets to ingest is smaller and may thus encourage patient adherence.

While there is ecological evidence of the benefits of FDCs in relation to drug resistance in early studies of DOTS programmes, there is limited direct evidence of improved adherence with FDCs (*4*). A recent multicentre trial found FDCs to have equivalent efficacy to single pills and to be more acceptable to patients (*5*). However, assessment of cure and relapses was based on smear microscopy and not on culture. A multicentre trial (The Union Study C) evaluating the efficacy, acceptability and toxicity of a four-drug FDC compared with loose pills given in the intensive phase of treatment has just been completed and results should soon be available. Another multicentre study including pharmacokinetic assessment is soon to be completed by WHO/TDR.

Quality assurance is essential to ensure adequate bioavailability of the component drugs of FDCs.[1] Using FDCs does not obviate the need for separate drugs for patients who develop drug toxicity or intolerance or for those with contraindications to specific component drugs.

3.3.2 Patient kits

A TB patient kit contains the full course of treatment for a single patient and thus assures the TB patient that his or her medicines will be available throughout treatment. The kit provides health workers with a container that has all required medicines in the necessary strengths and quantities. This helps limit confusion and wastage, and makes it easier to monitor the regularity of treatment; avoiding stock-outs also helps to maintain patient confidence in the health system. In addition, the patient may feel a sense of "ownership" of the patient kit and enhanced motivation to complete the full course of treatment – during visits to the health centre he or she can actually see the quantity of medicines that must be taken to achieve cure (1).

It should be noted that the TB patient kit does not eliminate the need for directly observed treatment (DOT).

3.4 Standard regimens for defined patient groups

Standardized treatment means that all patients in a defined group receive the same treatment regimen. Standard regimens have the following advantages over individualized prescription of drugs:

— errors in prescription – and thus the risk of development of drug resistance – are reduced;
— estimating drug needs, purchasing, distribution and monitoring are facilitated;
— staff training is facilitated;
— costs are reduced;
— maintaining a regular drug supply when patients move from one area to another is made easier;
— outcome evaluation is convenient and results are comparable.

For assigning standard regimens, patients are grouped by the same patient registration groups used for recording and reporting, which differentiate new patients from those who have had prior treatment. Registration groups for previously treated patients are based on the outcome of their prior treatment course: failure, relapse and default (see Chapter 2).

---

[1] See Global Drug Facility, www.stoptb.org/gdf/drugsupply/quality_sourcing_process.asp.

Recommended regimens for different patient registration groups are shown in Tables 3.2, 3.3 and 3.4. More details on the evidence and judgements underlying the recommended regimens are described in Annex 2.

3.5 New patients

New patients are defined as those who have no history of prior TB treatment or who received less than 1 month of anti-TB drugs (regardless of whether their smear or culture results are positive or not) (see section 2.6).

3.5.1 New patients presumed or known to have drug-susceptible TB

New patients are presumed to have drug-susceptible TB with two exceptions:

- Where there is a high prevalence of isoniazid resistance in new patients (see section 3.5.2).

  or

- If they have developed active TB after known contact with a patient documented to have drug-resistant TB; they are likely to have a similar drug resistance pattern to the source case (6), and DST should be carried out at the start of treatment. While DST results of the patient are awaited, a regimen based on the DST of the presumed source case should be started.

The 2-month rifampicin regimen (2HRZE/6HE) is associated with more relapses and deaths than the 6-month rifampicin regimen (2HRZE/4HR) (7). WHO therefore recommends the following for new patients presumed or known to have drug-susceptible TB. (See also Standard 8 of the ISTC (3).)

■ **Recommendation 1.1**
New patients with pulmonary TB should receive a regimen containing 6 months of rifampicin: 2HRZE/4HR

(Strong/High grade of evidence)

Remark a: Recommendation 1.1 also applies to extrapulmonary TB except TB of the central nervous system, bone or joint for which some expert groups suggest longer therapy (see Chapter 8).

Remark b: WHO recommends that national TB control programmes provide supervision and support for all TB patients in order to ensure completion of the full course of therapy.

Remark c: WHO recommends drug resistance surveys (or surveillance) for monitoring the impact of the treatment programme, as well as for designing standard regimens.

■ **Recommendation 1.2**
The 2HRZE/6HE treatment regimen should be phased out

(Strong/High grade of evidence)

In terms of dosing frequency for HIV-negative patients, the systematic review found little evidence of differences in failure or relapse rates with daily or three times weekly regimens (7). However, patients receiving three times weekly dosing throughout therapy had higher rates of acquired drug resistance than patients who received drugs daily throughout treatment. In patients with pre-treatment isoniazid resistance, three times weekly dosing during the intensive phase was associated with significantly higher risks of failure and acquired drug resistance than daily dosing during the intensive phase. (Treatment regimens for TB patients living with HIV are discussed in detail in Chapter 5.)

■ **Recommendation 2.1**
Wherever feasible, the optimal dosing frequency for new patients with pulmonary TB is daily throughout the course of therapy

(Strong/High grade of evidence)

There are two alternatives to Recommendation 2.1:

■ **Recommendation 2.1A**
New patients with pulmonary TB may receive a daily intensive phase followed by three times weekly continuation phase [2HRZE/4(HR)$_3$] provided that each dose is directly observed

(Conditional/High or moderate grade of evidence))

■ **Recommendation 2.1B**
Three times weekly dosing throughout therapy [2(HRZE)$_3$/4(HR)$_3$] is another alternative to Recommendation 2.1, provided that every dose is directly observed and the patient is NOT living with HIV or living in an HIV-prevalent setting

(Conditional/High or moderate grade of evidence))

Remark a: Treatment regimens for TB patients living with HIV or living in HIV-prevalent settings are discussed in Recommendation 4 and Chapter 5.

Remark b: In terms of dosing frequency for HIV-negative patients, the systematic review found little evidence of differences in failure or relapse rates with daily or three times weekly regimens (7). However, rates of acquired drug resistance were higher among patients receiving three times weekly dosing throughout therapy than among patients who received daily drug administration throughout treatment. Moreover, in patients with pretreatment isoniazid resistance, three times weekly dosing during the intensive phase was associated with significantly higher risks of failure and acquired drug resistance than daily dosing during the intensive phase.

There is insufficient evidence to support the efficacy of twice weekly dosing throughout therapy (7).

■ **Recommendation 2.2**

New patients with TB should not receive twice weekly dosing for the full course of treatment unless this is done in the context of formal research

(Strong/High grade of evidence)

Remark: The available evidence showed equivalent efficacy of daily intensive-phase dosing followed by two times weekly continuation phase (7). However, twice weekly dosing is not recommended on operational grounds, since missing one dose means the patient receives only half the regimen.

Tables 3.2a and 3.2b present standard treatment regimen and dosing frequency for new TB patients.

Table 3.2a STANDARD REGIMENS FOR NEW TB PATIENTS
(presumed, or known, to have drug-susceptible TB)

Intensive phase treatment	Continuation phase
2 months of HRZE[a]	4 months of HR

[a] WHO no longer recommends omission of ethambutol during the intensive phase of treatment for patients with non-cavitary, smear-negative PTB or EPTB who are known to be HIV-negative. In tuberculous meningitis, ethambutol should be replaced by streptomycin.

H = isoniazid, R = rifampicin, Z = pyrazinamide, E = ethambutol, S = streptomycin

Table 3.2b DOSING FREQUENCY FOR NEW TB PATIENTS

Dosing frequency		Comment
Daily	Daily	Optimal
Daily	Three times per week	Acceptable alternative for any new TB patient receiving directly observed therapy
Three times per week	Three times per week	Acceptable alternative provided that the patient is receiving directly observed therapy and is not living with HIV or living in an HIV-prevalent setting (See Chapter 5)

Note: Daily (rather than three times weekly) intensive-phase dosing may help to prevent acquired drug resistance in TB patients starting treatment with isoniazid resistance (see section 3.5.2).

3.5.2 Settings with high levels of isoniazid resistance in new patients

When new patients with isoniazid-resistant TB start their treatment, outcomes are worse than for patients with isoniazid-susceptible TB, even with the 6-month rifampicin regimen (7). The global weighted mean of any isoniazid resistance (excluding MDR) is 7.4% in new patients (8). Thus, a significant proportion of the new TB cases in many regions of the world have a risk of poor treatment outcomes because of their pretreatment isoniazid resistance.

The following weak recommendation applies to countries where isoniazid susceptibility testing in new patients is not done (or results are not available) before the continuation phase begins.

■ **Recommendation 3**

In populations with known or suspected high levels of isoniazid resistance, new TB patients may receive HRE as therapy in the continuation phase as an acceptable alternative to HR

(Weak/Insufficient evidence, expert opinion)

Given the potential benefit (9) and low risk of toxicity from ethambutol, the pressing need to prevent MDR warrants this recommendation. However, the recommendation is conditional, for the reasons explained in more detail in Annex 2. The most effective regimen for the treatment of isoniazid-resistant TB is not known. There is inadequate evidence to quantify the ability of ethambutol to "protect rifampicin" in patients with pre-treatment isoniazid resistance. The evidence for ocular toxicity from ethambutol was not systematically reviewed for this revision, but the risk of permanent blindness exists. Further research (see Annex 5) is therefore urgently needed to define the level of isoniazid resistance that would warrant the addition of ethambutol (or other drugs) to the continuation phase of the standard new patient regimen in TB programmes where isoniazid drug susceptibility testing is not done (or results are not available) before the continuation phase begins.

Daily (rather than three times weekly) intensive-phase dosing may also help to prevent acquired drug resistance in TB patients starting treatment with isoniazid resistance. The systematic review (7) found that patients with isoniazid resistance treated with a three times weekly intensive phase had significantly higher risks of failure and acquired drug resistance than those treated with daily dosing during the intensive phase.

Table 3.3 presents standard treatment regimens for new patients in settings with high isoniazid resistance.

Table 3.3   STANDARD REGIMENS FOR NEW TB PATIENTS
(in settings where the level of isoniazid resistance among new TB cases
is high and isoniazid susceptibility testing is not done (or results are not
available) before the continuation phase begins)

Intensive phase treatment	Continuation phase
2 months of HRZE	4 months of HRE

3.6 Previously treated patients and multidrug resistance

Previous TB treatment is a strong determinant of drug resistance (*10*), and previously treated patients comprise a significant proportion (13%) of the global TB notifications in 2007.

Of all the forms of drug resistance, it is most critical to detect multidrug resistance (MDR) because it makes regimens with first-line drugs much less effective (*11*) and resistance can be further amplified (*12*). Prompt identification of MDR and initiation of MDR treatment with second-line drugs gives a better chance of cure and prevents the development and spread of further resistance. Because of its clinical significance, MDR (rather than any drug resistance) is used to describe the retreatment patient groups below.

At the global level, 15% of previously treated patients have MDR (*8*), which is five times higher than the global average of 3% in new patients (Figure 3.1). Even in Africa, the WHO region thought to have the lowest level of MDR in retreatment patients, a significant proportion (6%) of retreatment patients have MDR-TB (*8*).[1] If their MDR is not detected and treated with second-line drugs, these patients will suffer poor outcomes and spread MDR in their communities.

WHO surveillance data from 10 countries found the level of MDR to be 32% in patients returning after defaulting or relapsing and significantly higher (49%) in patients whose prior treatment has failed (Figure 3.2).[2] Other studies show MDR levels of up to 80–90% in patients whose prior treatment courses have failed (*10–16*). Modelling described in Annex 2 predicts that, when a first course of treatment containing 6 months of rifampicin fails, 50–94% of patients have MDR-TB (compared with 4–56% of patients upon failure of a regimen containing 2 months of rifampicin).

Many factors influence the level of MDR in previously treated patients, and levels are likely to vary widely by setting. Assignment of the retreatment patient groups to medium vs high likelihood of MDR may therefore need to be modified according to country-specific data on similar groups of patients, as well as other factors discussed in section 3.8 below.

---

[1] Of 46 countries in Africa, 6 have reported drug resistance data since 2002; 22 countries (representing 72% of the region's cases) have reported data since 1994 (*5*, p. 90).

[2] These are the only 10 countries that reported drug resistance surveillance data by subcategory of retreatment cases since 1997.

Figure 3.1 WEIGHTED MEAN OF MDR-TB IN NEW AND RETREATMENT TB CASES FROM DRUG RESISTANCE SURVEYS, 1994–2007[a]

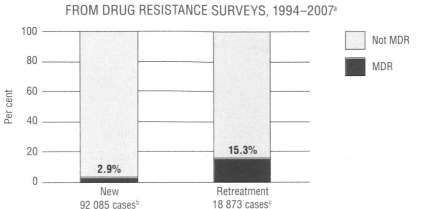

ᵃ Source: *Anti-tuberculosis drug resistance in the world: fourth global report.* Geneva, World Health Organization (2008) (*8*).
ᵇ Data from 105 countries or 127 settings.
ᶜ Data from 94 countries or 109 settings.

Figure 3.2 MDR IN RETREATMENT TB CASES FROM DRUG RESISTANCE SURVEYS AND SURVEILLANCE IN 10 COUNTRIES, 1997–2007[a]

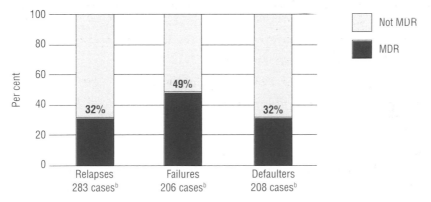

ᵃ Source: van Gemert W et al. *MDR among sub-categories of previously treated TB cases: an analysis in 12 settings.* Presented at: 40th World Conference on Lung Health, 3–7 December 2009, Cancun, Mexico.
ᵇ Data from 12 settings in 10 countries.

3.7 Standard regimens for previously treated patients

The *Global Plan to Stop TB 2006–2015* sets a target of all previously treated patients having access to DST at the beginning of treatment by 2015 (*17*). The purpose is to identify MDR as early as possible so that appropriate treatment can be given. (See also Standard 11 of the ISTC (*3*).)

■ **Recommendation 7.1**

Specimens for culture and drug susceptibility testing (DST) should be obtained from all previously treated TB patients at or before the start of treatment. DST should be performed for at least isoniazid and rifampicin

The approach to the initiation of retreatment depends on the country's laboratory capacity, specifically *when* (or if) DST results are routinely available for the individual patient. Countries using rapid molecular-based DST (*18*, *19*) will have results for rifampicin/isoniazid available within 1–2 days; these results can be used in deciding which regimen to start for the individual patient (section 3.7.1).

Using conventional DST methods yields results within weeks (for liquid media) or months (for solid media). Because of this delay, countries using conventional methods will need to start an empirical regimen while DST results are awaited. The choice of empirical retreatment regimens is discussed in section 3.7.2 below.

Where DST is not yet routinely available for individual retreatment patients, an interim approach could be implemented while the country is strengthening its laboratory system.

For many countries, drug resistance surveillance or surveys show that patients whose prior course of therapy has failed have a high likelihood of MDR (especially if the regimen contained 6 months of rifampicin, as described in Annex 2). Patients whose prior course of therapy has failed should therefore receive an empirical MDR regimen. Drug resistance surveillance or surveys often show that those relapsing or returning after default have a medium or low likelihood of MDR; such patients can receive the retreatment regimen of first-line drugs. However, levels of MDR in different patient registration groups vary by setting.[1]

It must be noted, however, that the retreatment regimen using first-line drugs is not supported by evidence deriving from clinical trials. It was designed primarily for use in settings with low prevalence of initial drug resistance and in patients previously treated with a regimen that included rifampicin for the first 2 months (*20*).

The assumption that patients whose treatment has failed have a high likelihood of MDR (and relapse or defaulting patients have a medium likelihood of MDR) may

---

[1] If drug resistance surveys show that patients relapsing or returning after default have high levels of MDR, they will need an MDR regimen instead. Similarly, if the country data show that levels of MDR are low in patients who failed their previous treatment, the NTP may decide to administer retreatment regimens with first-line drugs. See section 3.8 for further details.

need to be modified according to both the level of MDR found in these patient registration groups and the considerations discussed in section 3.8 (below).

Several other considerations (also described in section 3.8) will have an impact on the level of MDR the NTP designates as "high" in a given country. (See also Standard 12 of the ISTC (3).)

Countries will need to use a mix of approaches if they are in transition, where some areas of the country do not yet have DST results routinely available and others do, or some laboratories use rapid and others conventional DST methods.

3.7.1 Previously treated patients in settings with rapid DST

With line probe assays, MDR can be essentially confirmed[1] or excluded within 1–2 days,[2] which allows the results to guide the regimen at the start of therapy.

■ **Recommendation 7.2**
   In settings where rapid molecular-based DST is available, the results should guide the choice of regimen

The use of rapid molecular-based tests is discussed in more detail in section 3.8.1 below.

3.7.2 Previously treated patients in settings where conventional DST results are routinely available for individual patients

Obtaining specimens for conventional culture and DST should not delay the start of therapy. Empirical regimens, often based on drug-resistance surveillance data, are used while the results of conventional DST (liquid or solid media) are awaited, and should be started promptly.[3] This is especially important if the patient is seriously ill or the disease is progressing rapidly. Placing a patient on an empiric regimen pending DST is done to avoid clinical deterioration. Also, once empiric therapy begins to render the patient less infectious, the risk of transmission to contacts decreases.

While awaiting the results of conventional DST, WHO recommends administering an empiric MDR regimen[4] for patient groups with a high likelihood of MDR, and the retreatment regimen with first line drug regimen for patient groups with medium or low likelihood of MDR (Table 3.4).

---

[1] Line probe assays detect resistance to rifampicin alone or in combination with isoniazid resistance. Overall high accuracy for detection of MDR is retained when rifampicin resistance alone is used as a marker for MDR (19).

[2] From sputum samples or from bacterial cultures derived from those specimens.

[3] In some individual patients who have been treated multiple times, waiting to start treatment until DST results are available may be prudent provided that the patients are clinically stable and transmission to contacts is prevented. In most countries, however, adequate infection control measures are not yet in place.

[4] Guidance on designing a country's standard MDR regimen is provided in Chapter 7 of this document, and in Chapter 7 of *Guidelines for the programmatic management of drug-resistant TB* (6).

■ **Recommendation 7.3**

In settings where rapid molecular-based DST results are not routinely available to guide the management of individual patients, empiric treatment should be started as follows:

■ **Recommendation 7.3.1**

TB patients whose treatment has *failed*[1] or other patient groups with high likelihood of multidrug-resistant TB (MDR) should be started on an empirical MDR regimen

Remark a: In the absence of culture and DST results, the patient should be clinically evaluated before the MDR regimen is administered.

Remark b: Other examples of patients with high likelihood of MDR-TB are those relapsing or defaulting after their second or subsequent course of treatment. See also section 3.8.2.

■ **Recommendation 7.3.2**

TB patients returning after *defaulting* or *relapsing* from their first treatment course may receive the retreatment regimen containing first-line drugs 2HRZES/1HRZE/5HRE if country-specific data show low or medium levels of MDR in these patients or if such data are not available

Remark: When DST results become available, regimens should be adjusted appropriately.

3.7.3 Previously treated patients in settings where DST is not routinely available for individual patients

In the many countries that still lack the laboratory capacity to routinely conduct DST for each previously treated patient (or where results arrive too late to guide therapy), it is urgent to strengthen laboratory capacity. For countries without sufficient domestic funding, financial assistance is available from the Global Fund to Fight AIDS, Tuberculosis and Malaria, as well as from UNITAID or other international financing mechanisms. Technical assistance in laboratory strengthening is available from WHO, Global Laboratory Initiative and other partners.

Even though DST is not yet routinely available for individual patient management in these countries, the NTP may be able to collect or access some information on levels of MDR-TB in previously treated patients, by using data from a drug resistance survey, from a national or supranational reference laboratory, or from a referral or research centre (see section 3.8.2). These data are critical for ascertaining the level of

---

[1] Failures in a well-run NTP should be infrequent in the absence of MDR-TB. If they do occur, they are due either to MDR-TB or to programme factors such as poor DOT or poor drug quality. If drug resistance data from failure patients are available and these show low or medium levels of MDR, patients should receive the retreatment regimen outlined in 7.3.2, and every effort should be made to address the underlying programmatic issues.

MDR in retreatment patients.[1] For example, the results of representative drug resistance surveys may identify a group of patients among whom a very high percentage have MDR, which could justify the use of MDR regimens in all patients in the group (even if individual DST is not available) (6). The NTP manager is encouraged to obtain technical assistance from the Green Light Committee (see section 3.8.3).

If a very high level of MDR is documented in a specific group (such as patients who have failed a retreatment regimen), the NTP manager should urgently seek means to routinely obtain DST on all such patients at the start of treatment, in order to confirm or exclude MDR. If this cannot yet be achieved with any in-country laboratory, NTPs should make arrangements to send the specimens from these patients to a supranational reference or other international laboratory for DST while the country rapidly builds domestic laboratory capacity.

A country may face a short delay before a domestic or an international laboratory can perform DST on specimens from patients who are members of a group shown to have very high levels of MDR-TB. In these exceptional circumstances, an NTP may consider a short-term policy of directly starting such patients on an empirical MDR-TB regimen while awaiting confirmation of isoniazid and rifampicin resistance (last row of Table 3.4) (6). This is a *temporary measure* that can be implemented only if culture and DST can be arranged in the first few months of MDR treatment in each enrolled patient. It is essential to confirm the presence of MDR, and to monitor the response to treatment. (Groups of patients whose likelihood of MDR is medium or low will receive the 8-month retreatment regimen with first-line drugs.)

■ Recommendation 7.4

In settings where DST results are not yet routinely available to guide the management of individual patients, the empirical regimens will continue throughout the course of treatment

Remark: If DST results become available, regimens should be adjusted appropriately.

■ Recommendation 7.5

NTPs should obtain and use their country-specific drug resistance data on failure, relapse and default patient groups to determine the levels of MDR

Remark: Country-specific drug resistance data should include data stratified by type of regimen given for the patient's first course of TB treatment (i.e. 2 vs 6 months of rifampicin).

---

[1] This information is also needed to determine the patterns of MDR, so that a standard MDR regimen can be chosen for empirical treatment of patients with high likelihood of having MDR.

3.8 Overall considerations in selecting a country's standard regimens

National TB control programmes will need three standard regimens:

— "new patient regimen": the regimen containing 6 months of rifampicin: 2HRZE/4HR[1]
— "retreatment regimen with first-line drugs": 2HRZES/1HRZE/5HRE[2]
— "MDR regimen".

To implement these regimens in the country, the NTP needs to consider the following factors:

— availability of results of conventional or rapid molecular-based DST to guide management of individual patients;
— level of drug resistance in the country's new and previously treated patients;
— number of MDR-TB patients the programme has the capacity to enrol and treat;
— the short-term risk of dying from MDR-TB due to concomitant conditions (especially HIV, discussed in Chapter 5);
— availability of patient support and supervision (discussed in Chapter 6).

Many of these factors depend on available resources in the country, particularly the availability of DST and MDR-TB treatment. Because these essential elements of the Stop TB Strategy are not yet fully in place throughout the world, this chapter provides guidance on interim approaches.

Table 3.4 below presents suggestions for how the NTP manager can take account of these factors when selecting the standard regimens for defined patient groups.

3.8.1 Availability of DST results to guide management of individual patients: conventional and rapid methods

Ideally, DST is done for all patients at the start of treatment, so that the most appropriate therapy for each individual can be determined. However, the goal of universal access to DST has not yet been realized for most of the world's TB patients. While countries are expanding laboratory capacity and implementing new rapid tests (see below), WHO recommends that sputum specimens for testing susceptibility to isoniazid and rifampicin be obtained from the following patient groups at the start of treatment:

• All previously treated patients (*17, 21, 22*). The highest levels of MDR are found in patients whose prior course of therapy has failed (*6*).

• All persons living with HIV who are diagnosed with active TB, especially if they live in areas of moderate or high MDR prevalence. It is essential to detect MDR as soon as possible in persons living with HIV, given their high risk of mortality

---

[1] With or without ethambutol in the continuation phase (see section 3.5.2).
[2] Countries with rapid molecular-based DST will not need this regimen.

Table 3.4   STANDARD REGIMENS FOR PREVIOUSLY TREATED PATIENTS
depending on the availability of routine DST to guide the therapy of
individual retreatment patients

DST	Likelihood of MDR (patient registration group[a])	
Routinely available for previously treated patients	High (failure[b])	Medium or low (relapse, default)
Rapid molecular-based method	DST results available in 1–2 days confirm or exclude MDR to guide the choice of regimen	
Conventional method	While awaiting DST results:[c]	
	Empirical MDR regimen *Regimen should be modified once DST results are available.*	2HRZES/HRZE/5HRE *Regimen should be modified once DST results are available.*
None (interim)	Empirical MDR regimen *Regimen should be modified once DST results or DRS data are available.*	2HRZES/HRZE/5HRE for full course of treatment. *Regimen should be modified once DST results or DRS data are available.*

[a] The assumption that failure patients have a high likelihood of MDR (and relapse or defaulting patients a medium likelihood) may need to be modified according to the level of MDR in these patient registration groups, as well considerations discussed in section 3.8.

[b] And other patients in groups with high levels of MDR. One example is patients who develop active TB after known contact with a patient with documented MDR-TB. Patients who are relapsing or returning after defaulting from their second or subsequent course of treatment probably also have a high likelihood of MDR.

[c] Regimen may be modified once DST results are available (up to 2–3 months after the start of treatment).

Notes:

1. A country's standard MDR regimen is based on country-specific DST data from similar groups of patients (see Chapter 7).

2. In the country's standard regimens, the 8-month retreatment regimen should not be "augmented" by a fluoroquinolone or an injectable second-line drug; this practice jeopardizes second-line drugs that are critical treatment options for MDR patients. Second-line drugs should be used only for MDR regimens and only if quality-assured drugs can be provided by DOT for the whole course of therapy. In addition, there must be laboratory capacity for cultures to monitor treatment response, as well as a system for detecting and treating adverse reactions (see section 3.8.3 on the Green Light Committee Initiative) before embarking on MDR-TB treatment.

should they have MDR-TB. Some programmes recommend DST for HIV-infected TB patients with CD4 counts below 200 cells/mm³ (*6*).

- Persons who develop active TB after known exposure to a patient with documented MDR-TB.

- All new patients in countries where the level of MDR-TB in new patients is >3% (*23*).

In addition to the indications listed above for DST *at the start* of treatment (or re-treatment), WHO recommends that DST be performing *during* treatment in the following situation:

- New and previously treated patients who remain sputum smear-positive at the end of the intensive phase should submit another specimen for smear microscopy the following month. If that specimen is also smear-positive, culture and DST should be undertaken (see Recommendation 5.3 in Chapter 4). This will allow a result to be available earlier than the fifth month of treatment.

Comprehensive systems for managing the quality of laboratory services, including internal quality control and external quality assurance, are mandatory. Laboratories should follow standardized protocols for good laboratory practice, technical procedures and biosafety, in compliance with international standards (6). Documentary proof of sustained technical proficiency in DST is essential, and links with supranational TB reference laboratories to ensure DST quality are strongly encouraged. It is also important that appropriate specimens be obtained and rapidly transported to the laboratory. Because laboratory errors or discrepant results may occur, the clinical situation must be taken into account in interpreting the results of in vitro DST.

Conventional DST

WHO has endorsed the use of liquid culture and rapid species identification as preferable to solid culture-based methods alone. Liquid culture and rapid species identification should be based on a country-specific comprehensive plan for laboratory capacity strengthening and implemented in a step-wise manner. Liquid systems are more sensitive for detecting mycobacteria and may increase the case yield by 10% compared with solid media. Liquid systems may also yield DST results in as little as 10 days, compared with 28–42 days using conventional solid media.[1]

Longer delays in receiving DST results mean longer empirical treatment, which has significant disadvantages:

- With empirical use of the retreatment regimen with first-line drugs, patients whose DST eventually confirms MDR will have been inadequately treated while awaiting DST results. Consequences could include continued spread of MDR and amplification of resistance to include ethambutol.

- With empirical use of MDR regimens, patients whose DST eventually rules out MDR will have been exposed to toxic drugs they did not need while awaiting DST results. Consequences could include adverse drug effects and an increased risk of defaulting from treatment.

---

[1] See www.who.int/tb/dots/laboratory/policy/en/index3.html

Rapid DST

In contrast to conventional methods, molecular-amplification assays such as line probe assays allow detection of rifampicin resistance (alone or in combination with isoniazid) within days of sputum specimens being obtained from the patient (and can also be used on cultures obtained from rapid liquid culture systems). Patients with MDR-TB can avoid delays in starting an MDR regimen, and TB patients without MDR will avoid unnecessary second-line drug treatment. WHO strongly encourages the use of rapid molecular (and culture-based) DST in smear-positive persons living with HIV (6).

WHO recommends that ministries of health decide on line probe assays for rapid detection of MDR-TB within the context of country plans for appropriate management of MDR-TB patients; plans should also include the development of country-specific screening algorithms and timely access to quality-assured second-line anti-TB drugs (24).

Line probe assays have been adequately validated in direct testing of sputum smear-positive specimens, as well as on isolates of *M. tuberculosis* complex grown from smear-negative and smear-positive specimens. Direct use of line probe assays on smear-negative clinical specimens is not recommended. Adoption of line probe assays does not eliminate the need for conventional culture and DST capability; culture remains necessary for definitive diagnosis of TB in smear-negative patients, while conventional DST is required to determine drug susceptibility to drugs other than rifampicin and isoniazid. Additional guidance on selecting and implementing rapid drug susceptibility tests can be found on the WHO web site at: www.who.int/tb/features_archive/mdrtb_rapid_tests/en/index.html

3.8.2 Level of drug resistance in the country's new and previously treated patients

Countries reporting approximately half the world's TB cases have conducted at least one drug resistance survey since 1994 (8). These results, together with estimates of MDR-TB levels in all countries, are available on the WHO web site at: www.who.int/tb/features_archive/drsreport_launch_26feb08/en/index.html

New patients

Drug resistance information is critical for managing new patients and selecting the country's standard regimen for new patients:

- If country data (or WHO estimates) show that more than 3% of new patients have MDR, DST should be obtained at the start of therapy for all new patients (see section 3.8.1).

- Many countries have a high level of isoniazid resistance in new patients but do not have drug susceptibility results for isoniazid by the time of the continuation phase. In these countries, the NTP may select an isoniazid/rifampicin/ethambutol continuation phase for the standard regimen to be used for all new patients, as discussed in section 3.5.2.

Previously treated patients

As discussed in section 3.6 above, the NTP needs to review country-specific data to verify, or modify, the assignment of failure patients to high likelihood of MDR (Table 3.4) and patients returning after relapse or default to medium or low likelihood of MDR. Boxes 3.1, 3.2 and 3.3 provide examples of how these data may be used.

While WHO recommends that DST be performed on all previously treated cases (22), systems that will yield this critical information are not yet in place in most countries. Until countries have finished establishing the needed laboratory and surveillance capacity, information on the level of MDR in previously treated patients is available from a few other sources.

The Global Drug Resistance Surveillance project includes actual and estimated levels of MDR in previously treated patients as a whole, although sample sizes were usually too small to yield very precise estimates (8). Moreover, only 10 countries have measured MDR levels in subgroups of previously treated patients since 1994 (Figure 3.2).

Alternative sources of data are in-country laboratories, supranational reference laboratories, hospitals, treatment centres and research projects. The results must be interpreted with caution, as they represent only those patients who have accessed the specific services and those institutions where the testing is done. For example, the level of MDR found in a hospital-based survey in a capital city accepting referrals of the most difficult cases is likely to be higher than the level that would be found in unselected patients in a remote area.

BOX 3.1

AN EXAMPLE OF REASSIGNING PATIENT GROUPS BASED ON COUNTRY-SPECIFIC DRUG RESISTANCE SURVEY RESULTS

In Country A, a nationwide survey of all previously treated patients showed the following levels of MDR in patients:

- whose prior treatment failed: 90%
- who have relapsed: 85%
- returning after default: 30%

Because relapsing patients have nearly as high a level of MDR as those whose treatment has failed, Country A decides that relapsing patients (while awaiting their DST results) will receive the country's standard empirical MDR regimen. In the national version of Table 3.4 in its NTP manual, Country A moves relapse patients from medium to high likelihood of MDR so they are managed the same way as patients whose prior treatment has failed (while patients returning after default are treated with the 8-month retreatment regimen with first-line drugs).

Note on other patient-specific risk factors for MDR

By assigning registration groups of previously treated patients to high and medium likelihood of MDR, Table 3.4 incorporates Standard 11 of the ISTC (*3*). This standard recommends that an assessment of the likelihood of drug resistance be obtained for all patients at the start of treatment.

The most critical patient-specific risk factor for MDR-TB is prior TB treatment (*13, 14*).

Known contact with a proven MDR case is another important determinant and can be ascertained by TB programmes at the time of patient registration. Other TB patients observed to have elevated MDR levels in certain settings are those (*6*):

— treated in a programme that operates poorly;
— with a history of using anti-TB drugs of poor or unknown quality;
— who remain sputum smear-positive at month 2 or 3 of treatment (see Chapter 4);
— whose private-sector treatment has failed;
— exposed in institutions with an MDR outbreak or a high prevalence of MDR (such as certain prisons or mines);
— with co-morbid conditions associated with malabsorption or rapid-transit diarrhoea;
— living with HIV (in some settings);
— whose prior course of therapy included rifampicin throughout (Annex 2);
— have type 2 diabetes mellitus (*25*).

NTPs may be able to collect samples for DST from some of the patient groups listed above to determine their levels of MDR.

3.8.3 Number of MDR-TB patients the programme has the ca ̃ity to enrol

The Green Light Committee (GLC) Initiative helps countries to gain access to quality-assured second-line drugs[1] at considerably less than market prices. The GLC provides countries with high-level expertise in setting up and running MDR-TB programmes, integrated with routine TB control activities. Information about the GLC application process can be found online at: www.who.int/tb/challenges/mdr/greenlightcommittee/en/index.html

Projects intending to treat fewer than 50 patients can use a fast-track option to minimize the time required for the GLC application process. Countries with limited domestic resources for MDR detection and treatment can apply to the Global Fund to Fight AIDS, Tuberculosis and Malaria or other donors for funding.

---

[1] If second-line drugs are used, the NTP must ensure that they are quality-assured and can be provided by DOT throughout the entire 18–24 months it takes to treat MDR TB. In addition, laboratory capacity to monitor response to treatment and a system for detecting and treating adverse reactions must be in place.

BOX 3.2

AN EXAMPLE OF ASSIGNING THE PATIENT GROUP WITH THE HIGHEST MDR LEVELS TO RECEIVE EMPIRICAL MDR TREATMENT, AND LATER ADDING A PATIENT GROUP WITH THE NEXT HIGHEST MDR LEVELS, DURING SCALE-UP OF MDR-TB TREATMENT

Based on a special survey in one province, Country B finds an MDR level of 90% in TB patients whose treatment failed after two or more prior courses. For patients whose first treatment course failed, the level is 60%. The TB patients in this province are roughly representative of the whole country's TB patients. In Country B, DST of isoniazid and rifampicin is done routinely for individual patients whose previous treatment has failed but results are typically not available for 4 months.

Country B has just begun a Green Light Committee Initiative project and has the capacity to treat a very limited number of MDR-TB patients. It recommends that patients whose second or subsequent course of treatment has failed be managed as patients with a high likelihood of MDR (as recommended in Table 3.4) and receive an empirical regimen for MDR while DST results are awaited. Until the MDR programme is scaled up further, patients whose first treatment course has failed will be managed as those with a medium likelihood of MDR. Empirically, they all start the retreatment regimen with first-line drugs. When DST results are available 4 months later, those confirmed as having MDR-TB are changed to the MDR regimen.

Two years later, another drug resistance survey continues to show that 60% of patients whose first treatment failed have MDR, and their outcomes have been poor when treated empirically with the retreatment regimen of first-line drugs for the 4 months it takes to obtain DST results. By contrast, treatment with the country's standard MDR regimen is having good success in the patients in whom two or more prior treatment courses have failed. The country applies for and receives additional support from the Global Fund to now use empirical MDR regimens (while awaiting DST results) for patients whose first treatment course has failed.

As sufficient funding becomes available, countries will provide universal access to MDR-TB treatment. The stage of implementation has a bearing on the level of MDR that the country will use to define "high", "medium" and "low" likelihood of MDR.

At the beginning of an MDR programme, when the availability of MDR treatment is very limited, the NTP may chose to include only the very highest risk patients in the "high likelihood of MDR" group for empirical MDR treatment while DST results are awaited. As the programme is scaled up, the NTP manager can include more patients who need MDR treatment. Thus, there are no absolute thresholds for low, moderate, or high likelihood or levels of MDR: NTP managers will define them for their own country and will need to redefine them as progress is made towards universal access to MDR-TB treatment.

BOX 3.3

AN EXAMPLE OF WEIGHING THE HARMS AND BENEFITS OF EMPIRICAL MDR TREATMENT IN A SETTING OF HIGH HIV PREVALENCE

In Country C, 80% of all TB patients are living with HIV, and 30% of relapse patients have MDR. While the country is planning to implement rapid DST, it takes an average of 2 months to obtain results using the current conventional methods. The NTP is deciding which empirical regimen to include in the NTP manual for relapse patients for the 2 months it takes to obtain DST results.

Given the high level of HIV and the attendant risks of early death from untreated MDR-TB, the NTP decides to recommend that all relapse patients be treated with the country's empirical MDR regimen while DST results are awaited. The benefit of preventing early deaths in the 30% of relapse patients who *do* have MDR is judged to be greater than the possible harms[a] of MDR treatment (during the 2 months awaiting DST results) in the 70% of relapse patients who will prove to *not* have MDR.

[a] Possible harms include drug toxicity, increased likelihood of patient default, and burden on patient and programme resources.

3.8.4   Short-term risk of death from MDR-TB

Clinicians faced with a very ill TB patient suspected of having MDR-TB will initiate an MDR regimen while DST results are pending, even if the likelihood of MDR may be intermediate rather than high. The clinician judges that the risk of toxicity of the MDR regimen is outweighed by the possible life-saving benefit of the MDR regimen.

Similar judgements apply to regimen decisions at the level of the NTP. If previously treated patients as a group have frequent concomitant conditions (such as HIV) that increase the risk of short-term death from MDR-TB, the NTP will want to recommend an empirical MDR regimen for more retreatment patients while DST results are awaited. (WHO also recommends the use of rapid molecular-based tests in smear-positive persons found to be living with HIV, as well as culture-based DST to determine additional drug susceptibility (6).)

3.8.5 Availability of patient support and supervision

The availability of good quality patient support and supervision is essential to implementation of the regimens recommended in this chapter. The importance of the capacity of TB programmes to provide patient-centred care is discussed in Chapter 6.

References

1. Rational Pharmaceutical Management Plus Program. *Managing pharmaceuticals and commodities for tuberculosis: a guide for national tuberculosis programs.* Arlington, VA, Management Sciences for Health, 2005.

2. American Thoracic Society, CDC, Infectious Diseases Society of America. Treatment of tuberculosis. *Morbidity and Mortality Weekly Report: Recommendations and Reports*, 2003, 52(RR-11):1–77.

3. *International Standards for Tuberculosis Care (ISTC)*, 2nd ed. The Hague, Tuberculosis Coalition for Technical Assistance, 2009.

4. Connor J, Rafter N, Rodgers A. Do fixed-dose combination pills or unit-of-use packaging improve adherence? A systematic review. *Bulletin of the World Health Organization*, 2004, 82:935–939.

5. Bartacek A et al. Comparison of a four-drug fixed-dose combination regimen with a single tablet regimen in smear-positive pulmonary tuberculosis. *International Journal of Tuberculosis and Lung Disease*, 2009, 13:760–766.

6. *Guidelines for the programmatic management of drug-resistant tuberculosis: emergency update 2008.* Geneva, World Health Organization, 2008 (WHO/HTM/TB/2008.402).

7. Menzies D et al. Effect of duration and intermittency of rifampin on tuberculosis treatment outcomes: a systematic review and meta-analysis. *PloS Medicine*, 2009, 6:e1000146.

8. *Anti-tuberculosis drug resistance in the world: fourth global report.* Geneva, World Health Organization, 2008 (WHO/HTM/TB/2008.394).

9. Mitchison DA. Basic mechanisms of chemotherapy. *Chest*, 1979, 76(6 Suppl.): 771–781.

10. Espinal MA et al. Determinants of drug-resistant tuberculosis: analysis of 11 countries. *International Journal of Tuberculosis and Lung Disease*, 2001, 5:887–893.

11. Espinal MA et al. Standard short-course chemotherapy for drug-resistant tuberculosis: treatment outcomes in 6 countries. *Journal of the American Medical Association*, 2000, 283:2537–2545.

12. Quy HT et al. Drug resistance among failure and relapse cases of tuberculosis: is the standard re-treatment regimen adequate? *International Journal of Tuberculosis and Lung Disease*, 2003, 7:631–636.

13. Saravia JC et al. Retreatment management strategies when first-line tuberculosis therapy fails. *International Journal of Tuberculosis and Lung Disease*, 2005, 9:421–429.

14. Yoshiyama T et al. Development of acquired drug resistance in recurrent tuberculosis patients with various previous treatment outcomes. *International Journal of Tuberculosis and Lung Disease*, 2004, 8:31–38.

15. Drobniewski F et al. Drug-resistant tuberculosis, clinical virulence, and the dominance of the Beijing strain family in Russia. *Journal of the American Medical Association*, 2005, 293:2726–2731.

16. Faustini A, Hall AJ, Perucci CA. Risk factors for multidrug resistant tuberculosis in Europe: a systematic review. *Thorax*, 2006, 61:158–163.

17. *The Global Plan to Stop TB, 2006–2015.* Geneva, World Health Organization, 2006 (WHO/HTM/STB/2006.35).

18. Barnard M et al. Rapid molecular screening for multidrug-resistant tuberculosis in a high-volume public health laboratory in South Africa. *American Journal of Respiratory and Critical Care Medicine*, 2008, 177:787–792.

19. Sam IC et al. Mycobacterium tuberculosis and rifampin resistance, United Kingdom. *Emerging Infectious Diseases*, 2006, 12:752–759.

20. Menzies D et al. Standardized treatment of active tuberculosis in patients with previous treatment and/or with mono-resistance to isoniazid: a systematic review and meta-analysis. *PloS Medicine*, 2009, 6:e1000150.

21. *The global MDR-TB & XDR-TB response plan 2007–2008.* Geneva, World Health Organization, 2007 (WHO/HTM/TB/2007.387).

22. *Guidelines for the surveillance of drug resistance in tuberculosis*, 4th ed. Geneva, World Health Organization, 2009 (WHO/HTM/TB/2009.422).

23. Espinal M, Raviglione MC. From threat to reality: the real face of multidrug-resistant tuberculosis. *American Journal of Respiratory and Critical Care Medicine*, 2008, 178:216–217.

24. *Molecular line probe assays for rapid screening of patients at risk of MDR TB: policy statement.* Geneva, World Health Organization, 2008 (available at: www.who.int/tb/features_archive/policy_statement.pdf).

25. Fisher-Hoch SP et al. Type 2 diabetes and multidrug-resistant tuberculosis. *Scandinavian Journal of Infectious Diseases*, 2008, 40:888–893.

Monitoring during treatment

4.1 Chapter objectives

This chapter describes how to:

— monitor and record the response to treatment, and decide on actions to take in response to monitoring results;
— use cohort analysis to evaluate treatment outcomes;
— manage treatment interruption;
— detect and manage drug-induced toxicity.

4.2 Monitoring the patient

All patients should be monitored to assess their response to therapy (Standard 10 of the ISTC (*1*)). Regular monitoring of patients also facilitates treatment completion and allows the identification and management of adverse drug reactions. All patients, their treatment supporters and health workers should be instructed to report the persistence or reappearance of symptoms of TB (including weight loss), symptoms of adverse drug reactions, or treatment interruptions.

Patient weight should be monitored each month, and dosages should be adjusted if weight changes. Additional monitoring and the actions it triggers are discussed below for pulmonary and extrapulmonary cases treated with first-line drugs. For monitoring of patients receiving second-line drugs, see Chapter 7.

A written record of all medications given, bacteriological response and adverse reactions should be maintained for every patients on the TB Treatment Card (*2*) (Standard 13 of the ISTC (*1*)).

4.3 Assessing treatment response in new and previously treated pulmonary TB patients, and acting on the results

Response to treatment in pulmonary TB patients is monitored by sputum smear examination (see Figures 4.1 and 4.2 below).

■ **Recommendation 5.1**

For smear-positive pulmonary TB patients treated with first-line drugs, sputum smear microscopy may be performed at completion of the intensive phase of treatment

(Conditional/High or moderate grade of evidence)

Figure 4.1 SPUTUM MONITORING BY SMEAR MICROSCOPY IN NEW PULMONARY TB PATIENTS

Note: If a patient is found to harbour a multidrug-resistant strain of TB at any time during therapy, treatment is declared a failure and the patient is re-registered and should be referred to an MDR-TB treatment programme.

Months of treatment					
1	**2**	**3**	**4**	**5**	**6**
[========	========]	[---------------	----------------	----------------	---------------]
	•			•[a]	•[a]
				if sm +, obtain culture, DST[b]	if sm +, obtain culture, DST[b]

If smear-positive at month 2, obtain sputum again at month 3. If smear-positive at month 3, obtain culture and DST.

1	**2**	**3**	**4**	**5**	**6**
[========	========]	[---------------	----------------	----------------	---------------]
	•	•		•	•
	(sm +)	if sm +, obtain culture, DST		if sm +, obtain culture, DST[b]	if sm +, obtain culture, DST[b]

Key:
[========] Intensive phase of treatment (HRZE)
[------------] Continuation phase (HR)
• Sputum smear examination
sm + Smear-positive
[a] Omit if patient was smear-negative at the start of treatment and at 2 months.
[b] Smear- or culture-positivity at the fifth month or later (or detection of MDR-TB at any point) is defined as treatment failure and necessitates re-registration and change of treatment as described in section 3.7.

Figure 4.2 SPUTUM MONITORING OF PULMONARY TB PATIENTS RECEIVING THE 8-MONTH RETREATMENT REGIMEN WITH FIRST-LINE DRUGS

Months of treatment							
1	**2**	**3**	**4**	**5**	**6**	**7**	**8**
[========	========	========]	[--------------	---------------	----------------	----------------	-------------]
		•		•			•
		if sm +, obtain culture, DST		if sm +, obtain culture, DST[a]			if sm +, obtain culture, DST[a]

Key:
[========] Intensive phase: 2 months of HRZES followed by 1 month of HRZE
[------------] Continuation phase with 5 months of HRE
• Sputum smear examination
sm + Smear-positive
[a] Smear- or culture-positivity at the fifth month or later (or detection of MDR-TB at any point) is defined as treatment failure and necessitates reregistration and change of treatment as described in section 3.7.

This recommendation applies both to new patients treated with regimens containing 6 months of rifampicin (2HRZE/4HR) and to previously treated patients receiving the 8-month retreatment regimen with first-line drugs (2HRZES/1HRZE/5HRE). Sputum should be collected when the patient is given the last dose of the intensive-phase treatment. The end of the intensive phase is at 2 months in new patients and 3 months in previously treated patients receiving the 8-month regimen of first-line drugs. This recommendation also applies to smear-negative patients.

Sputum specimens should be collected for smear examination at each follow-up sputum check. They should be collected without interrupting treatment and transported to the laboratory as soon as possible thereafter; if a delay is unavoidable, specimens should be refrigerated or kept in as cool a place as possible.

Smear status at the end of the intensive phase is a poor predictor of which new patients will relapse.[1] However, detection of a positive sputum smear remains important as a trigger for the patient assessment outlined below as well as for additional sputum monitoring described in sections 4.3.1 and 4.3.2. The proportion of smear-positive patients with sputum smear conversion at the end of the intensive phase is also an indicator of TB programme performance.

A positive sputum smear at the end of the intensive phase may indicate any of the following:

— the initial phase of therapy was poorly supervised and patient adherence was poor;
— poor quality of anti-TB drugs;
— doses of anti-TB drugs are below the recommended range;
— resolution is slow because the patient had extensive cavitation and a heavy initial bacillary load;
— there are co-morbid conditions that interfere either with adherence or with response;
— the patient may have drug-resistant *M. tuberculosis* that is not responding to first-line treatment;
— non-viable bacteria remain visible by microscopy (3).

The programme should carefully review the quality of the patient's support and supervision and intervene promptly if necessary. Patient treatment records should be reviewed with the responsible health care worker, and reasons for any interruptions should be explored and addressed (4).

It is unnecessary, unreliable and wasteful of resources to monitor the patient by chest radiography.

---

[1] Systematic review was not published by the time of publication of this document. GRADE tables are available from WHO upon request.

4.3.1   New pulmonary TB patients

Additional sputum monitoring is needed for new patients whose sputum smear is positive at the end of the intensive phase (Standard 10 of the ISTC (*1*)).

■ **Recommendation 5.2**

In new patients, if the specimen obtained at the end of the intensive phase (month 2) is smear-positive, sputum smear microscopy should be obtained at the end of the third month

(Strong/High grade of evidence)

■ **Recommendation 5.3**

In new patients, if the specimen obtained at the end of month 3 is smear-positive, sputum culture and drug susceptibility testing (DST) should be performed

(Strong/High grade of evidence)

The main purpose of obtaining cultures at this stage is to detect drug resistance without waiting until the fifth month to change to appropriate therapy.[1] (Note that treatment is declared a failure if a patient is found to harbour MDR-TB at any point in time during treatment; see Table 4.1.)

If the country does not yet have sufficient laboratory capacity for culture and DST, additional monitoring of patients who are still smear-positive at month 3 will be only by sputum smear microscopy during the fifth month and during the final month of treatment. If either result is positive, treatment has failed, the patient is reregistered and treatment is changed as described in Chapter 3.

New pulmonary TB patients with positive sputum smears at the start of treatment
These patients should be monitored by sputum smear microscopy at the end of the fifth and sixth months. If results at the fifth or sixth month are positive, a sputum specimen should be obtained for culture and DST. Treatment has failed, the TB Treatment Card is closed (Outcome = treatment failure) and a new one is opened (Type of patient = treatment after failure). Treatment should follow the recommendations in Chapter 3. If a patient is found to harbour a multidrug-resistant strain of TB at any point of time during therapy, treatment is also declared a failure. See Figure 4.1 for a monitoring scheme with sputum smear microscopy.

New pulmonary TB patients whose sputum smear microscopy was negative
(or not done) at the start of treatment
It is important to recheck a sputum specimen at the end of the intensive phase in case of disease progression (due to non-adherence or drug resistance) or an error at the time of initial diagnosis (i.e. a true smear-positive patient was misdiagnosed

---

[1]   Even if there is eventually full susceptibility, a positive culture confirms poor response to treatment, which necessitates investigation and intervention.

as smear-negative).[1] Pulmonary TB patients whose sputum smear microscopy was negative (or not done) before treatment and whose sputum smears are negative at 2 months need no further sputum monitoring. They should be monitored clinically; body weight is a useful progress indicator.

4.3.2 Previously treated sputum smear-positive pulmonary TB patients receiving first-line anti-TB drugs

Sputum smear examination is performed at the end of the intensive phase of treatment (the 3rd month), at the end of the fifth month and at the end of treatment (the eighth month). If the country has already developed sufficient laboratory capacity, culture and DST should be performed at the start of treatment and, if smears are positive, at any of these points in time. See Figure 4.2 for a monitoring scheme with sputum smear microscopy.

■ **Recommendation 5.4**

   In previously treated patients, if the specimen obtained at the end of the intensive phase (month 3) is smear-positive, sputum culture and drug susceptibility testing (DST) should be performed

   (Strong/High grade of evidence)

4.4 Extrapulmonary TB

For patients with extrapulmonary TB, clinical monitoring is the usual way of assessing the response to treatment (Standard 10 of the ISTC (*1*)). As in pulmonary smear-negative disease, the weight of the patient is a useful indicator.

4.5 Recording standardized treatment outcomes

At the end of the treatment course for each individual patient, the District TB Officer records the treatment outcome in the District TB Register. Table 4.1 shows the definitions of standardized treatment outcomes.

4.6 Cohort analysis of treatment outcomes

A cohort is a group of patients diagnosed and registered for treatment during a specific time period (usually one-quarter of a year). Evaluation of treatment outcome in new pulmonary smear-positive patients is used as a major indicator of programme quality. Outcomes in other patients (retreatment, pulmonary smear-negative, extrapulmonary) are analysed in separate cohorts. (For guidance on cohort analysis of MDR-TB patients, see reference 5.)

Cohort analysis is the key management tool used to evaluate the effectiveness of the national TB control programme. It enables the identification of problems, so that the

---

[1]   If the sputum is found to be smear-positive, see Recommendations 5.2 and 5.3 above.

programme managers and staff can institute appropriate action to overcome them and improve programme performance. Evaluation of the outcomes of treatment and trends must be done at peripheral, district, regional and national levels to allow any necessary corrective action to be taken. It can also identify districts or units that are performing well and allows for positive feedback to be provided to staff; successful practices can then be replicated elsewhere.

Table 4.1   DEFINITIONS OF TREATMENT OUTCOMES[a]

Outcome	Definition
Cure	A patient whose sputum smear or culture was positive at the beginning of the treatment but who was smear- or culture-negative in the last month of treatment and on at least one previous occasion.
Treatment completed	A patient who completed treatment but who does not have a negative sputum smear or culture result in the last month of treatment and on at least one previous occasion[b]
Treatment failure	A patient whose sputum smear or culture is positive at 5 months or later during treatment. Also included in this definition are patients found to harbour a multidrug-resistant (MDR) strain at any point of time during the treatment, whether they are smear-negative or -positive.
Died	A patient who dies for any reason during the course of treatment.
Default	A patient whose treatment was interrupted for 2 consecutive months or more.
Transfer out	A patient who has been transferred to another recording and reporting unit and whose treatment outcome is unknown.
Treatment success	A sum of cured and completed treatment[c]

[a] These definitions apply to pulmonary smear-positive and smear-negative patients, and to patients with extrapulmonary disease. Outcomes in these patients need to be evaluated separately.
[b] The sputum examination may not have been done or the results may not be available.
[c] For smear- or culture-positive patients only.

The district/local TB officer should perform cohort analysis of treatment outcome every quarter-year and at the end of every year. A typical cohort consists of all TB patients registered during a quarter. New patients and subcategories of previously treated patients (relapses, return after default, failures) should be analysed as separate cohorts because they have different characteristics and expected results. Evaluation of outcome at the end of treatment should be undertaken as soon as possible after the last patient in the cohort completes treatment.[1]

This information is transmitted in quarterly reports. After local review, district re-

---

[1] Outcomes are routinely evaluated at the beginning of the quarter following the completion of treatment by the last patient in that cohort.

ports on treatment outcome are forwarded to the region each quarter. The regional/ intermediate TB officer should verify that district reports are correct, complete and consistent, compile cohort analysis reports on the sputum smear-positive patients in the region, and submit the report to the central unit of the NTP. The NTP compiles cohort analysis reports on the smear-positive TB patients registered nationally, evaluates, and provides feedback to the programme staff.

4.7 Management of treatment interruption

Supporting patients to prevent treatment interruption is discussed in Chapter 6; this section covers what to do if treatment is interrupted.

If a patient misses an arranged appointment to receive treatment, the NTP should ensure that the patient is contacted within a day after missing treatment during the initial phase, and within a week during the continuation phase. The patient can be traced using the locating information previously obtained (see section 6.5) (6). It is important to find out the cause of the patient's absence so that appropriate action can be taken and treatment can continue.

The management of patients who have interrupted treatment takes into consideration several factors, each of which, if present, will necessitate further caution and probably additional treatment (7):

- The patient is found to be smear- or culture-positive upon returning from default.
- Interruption occurs in the intensive, rather than the continuation, phase.
- Interruption occurs early (rather than later) in the continuation phase.
- The interruption is of long duration.
- The patient is immunocompromised (living with HIV or another condition).
- The patient had poor response to treatment before the interruption.
- Drug-resistant disease is known or suspected.

Culture and DST should be performed upon return of patients who meet the definition in Table 4.1 for default (interrupted treatment for at least 2 consecutive months). If laboratory capacity permits, specimens for culture and DST should also be obtained from other patients returning after treatment interruption.

4.8 Prevention of adverse effects of drugs

Health personnel can prevent some drug-induced side-effects, for example isoniazid-induced peripheral neuropathy. This usually presents as numbness or a tingling or burning sensation of the hands or feet and occurs more commonly in pregnant women and in people with the following conditions: HIV infection, alcohol dependency, malnutrition, diabetes, chronic liver disease, renal failure. These patients should receive preventive treatment with pyridoxine, 10 mg/day along with their anti-TB drugs. (Other guidelines recommend 25 mg/day (7).)

4.9 Monitoring and recording adverse effects

Most TB patients complete their treatment without any significant adverse drug effects. However, a few patients do experience adverse effects. It is therefore important that patients be clinically monitored during treatment so that adverse effects can be detected promptly and managed properly. Routine laboratory monitoring is not necessary.

Health personnel can monitor adverse drug effects by teaching patients how to recognize the symptoms of common effects, urging them to report if they develop such symptoms, and by asking about symptoms when patients come to collect drugs.

Adverse reactions to drugs should be recorded on the TB Treatment Card under "Observations".

Monitoring of patients receiving second-line drugs is covered in Chapter 7.

4.10 Symptom-based approach to managing side-effects of anti-TB drugs

The adverse effects of essential anti-TB drugs are described in Annex 1. Table 4.2 shows a symptom-based approach to the management of the most common adverse effects, which effects are classified as major or minor. In general, a patient who develops minor adverse effects should continue the TB treatment and be given symptomatic treatment. If a patient develops a major side-effect, the treatment or the responsible drug is stopped; the patient should be urgently referred to a clinician or health care facility for further assessment and treatment. Patients with major adverse reactions should be managed in a hospital.

4.10.1 Management of cutaneous reactions

If a patient develops itching without a rash and there is no other obvious cause, the recommended approach is to try symptomatic treatment with antihistamines and skin moisturizing, and continue TB treatment while observing the patient closely. If a skin rash develops, however, all anti-TB drugs must be stopped.

Once the reaction has resolved, anti-TB drugs are reintroduced one by one, starting with the drug least likely to be responsible for the reaction (rifampicin or isoniazid) at a small challenge dose, such as 50 mg isoniazid (3). The dose is gradually increased over 3 days. This procedure is repeated, adding in one drug at a time. A reaction after adding in a particular drug identifies that drug as the one responsible for the reaction. The alternative regimens listed in section 4.10.2 below are also applicable when a particular drug cannot be used because it was implicated as the cause of a cutaneous reaction.

4.10.2 Management of drug-induced hepatitis

This section covers hepatitis presumed to be induced by TB treatment. (For a discussion of TB treatment in patients with underlying liver disease, see Chapter 8.)

Table 4.2   SYMPTOM-BASED APPROACH TO MANAGING SIDE-EFFECTS
OF ANTI-TB DRUGS

Side-effects	Drug(s) probably responsible	Management
Major		*Stop responsible drug(s) and refer to clinician urgently*
Skin rash with or without itching	Streptomycin, isoniazid, rifampicin, pyrazinamide	Stop anti-TB drugs
Deafness (no wax on otoscopy)	Streptomycin	Stop streptomycin
Dizziness (vertigo and nystagmus)	Streptomycin	Stop streptomycin
Jaundice (other causes excluded), hepatitis	Isoniazid, pyrazinamide, rifampicin	Stop anti-TB drugs
Confusion (suspect drug-induced acute liver failure if there is jaundice)	Most anti-TB drugs	Stop anti-TB drugs
Visual impairment (other causes excluded)	Ethambutol	Stop ethambutol
Shock, purpura, acute renal failure	Rifampicin	Stop rifampicin
Decreased urine output	Streptomycin	Stop streptomycin
Minor		*Continue anti-TB drugs, check drug doses*
Anorexia, nausea, abdominal pain	Pyrazinamide, rifampicin, isoniazid	Give drugs with small meals or just before bedtime, and advise patient to swallow pills slowly with small sips of water. If symptoms persist or worsen, or there is protracted vomiting or any sign of bleeding, consider the side-effect to be major and refer to clinician urgently.
Joint pains	Pyrazinamide	Aspirin or non-steroidal anti-inflammatory drug, or paracetamol
Burning, numbness or tingling sensation in the hands or feet	Isoniazid	Pyridoxine 50–75 mg daily (3)
Drowsiness	Isoniazid	Reassurance. Give drugs before bedtime
Orange/red urine	Rifampicin	Reassurance. Patients should be told when starting treatment that this may happen and is normal
Flu syndrome (fever, chills, malaise, headache, bone pain)	Intermittent dosing of rifampicin	Change from intermittent to daily rifampicin administration (3)

Of the first-line anti-TB drugs, isoniazid, pyrazinamide and rifampicin can all cause liver damage (drug-induced hepatitis). In addition, rifampicin can cause asymptomatic jaundice without evidence of hepatitis. It is important to try to rule out other possible causes before deciding that the hepatitis is induced by the TB regimen.

The management of hepatitis induced by TB treatment depends on:

— whether the patient is in the intensive or continuation phase of TB treatment;
— the severity of the liver disease;
— the severity of the TB; and
— the capacity of the health unit to manage the side-effects of TB treatment.

If it is thought that the liver disease is caused by the anti-TB drugs, all drugs should be stopped. If the patient is severely ill with TB and it is considered unsafe to stop TB treatment, a non-hepatotoxic regimen consisting of streptomycin, ethambutol and a fluoroquinolone should be started.

If TB treatment has been stopped, it is necessary to wait for liver function tests to revert to normal and clinical symptoms (nausea, abdominal pain) to resolve before reintroducing the anti-TB drugs. If it is not possible to perform liver function tests, it is advisable to wait an extra 2 weeks after resolution of jaundice and upper abdominal tenderness before restarting TB treatment. If the signs and symptoms do not resolve and the liver disease is severe, the non-hepatotoxic regimen consisting of streptomycin, ethambutol and a fluoroquinolone should be started (or continued) for a total of 18–24 months (7).

Once drug-induced hepatitis has resolved, the drugs are reintroduced one at a time. If symptoms recur or liver function tests become abnormal as the drugs are reintroduced, the last drug added should be stopped. Some advise starting with rifampicin because it is less likely than isoniazid or pyrazinamide to cause hepatotoxicity and is the most effective agent (7, 8). After 3–7 days, isoniazid may be reintroduced. In patients who have experienced jaundice but tolerate the reintroduction of rifampicin and isoniazid, it is advisable to avoid pyrazinamide.

Alternative regimens depend on which drug is implicated as the cause of the hepatitis.

If rifampicin is implicated, a suggested regimen without rifampicin is 2 months of isoniazid, ethambutol and streptomycin followed by 10 months of isoniazid and ethambutol.

If isoniazid cannot be used, 6–9 months of rifampicin, pyrazinamide and ethambutol can be considered.

If pyrazinamide is discontinued before the patient has completed the intensive phase, the total duration of isoniazid and rifampicin therapy may be extended to 9 months (7).

If neither isoniazid nor rifampicin can be used, the non-hepatotoxic regimen consisting of streptomycin, ethambutol and a fluoroquinolone should be continued for a total of 18–24 months.

Reintroducing one drug at a time is the optimal approach, especially if the patient's hepatitis was severe. National TB control programmes using FDC tablets should therefore stock limited quantities of single anti-TB drugs for use in such cases. However, if the country's health units do not yet have single anti-TB drugs, clinical experience in resource-limited settings has been successful with the following approach, which depends on whether the hepatitis with jaundice occurred during the intensive or the continuation phase.

- *When hepatitis with jaundice occurs during the intensive phase* of TB treatment with isoniazid, rifampicin, pyrazinamide and ethambutol: once hepatitis has resolved, restart the same drugs EXCEPT replace pyrazinamide with streptomycin to complete the 2-month course of initial therapy, followed by rifampicin and isoniazid for the 6-month continuation phase.

- *When hepatitis with jaundice occurs during the continuation phase:* once hepatitis has resolved, restart isoniazid and rifampicin to complete the 4-month continuation phase of therapy.

References

1. *International Standards for Tuberculosis Care (ISTC)*, 2nd ed. The Hague, Tuberculosis Coalition for Technical Assistance, 2009.
2. *Revised TB recording and reporting forms and registers – version 2006*. Geneva, World Health Organization, 2006 (WHO/HTM/TB/2006.373; available at: http://www. who.int/tb/dots/r_and_r_forms/en/index.html).
3. Toman K. *Toman's tuberculosis. Case detection, treatment, and monitoring: questions and answers*, 2nd ed. Geneva, World Health Organization, 2004.
4. Williams G et al. *Best practice of the care for patients with tuberculosis: a guide for low income countries*. Paris, International Union Against Tuberculosis and Lung Disease, 2007.
5. *Guidelines for the programmatic management of drug-resistant tuberculosis: emergency update 2008*. Geneva, World Health Organization, 2008 (WHO/HTM/TB/2008.402).
6. Williams G et al. Care during the intensive phase: promotion of adherence. *International Journal of Tuberculosis and Lung Disease*, 2008, 12:601–605.
7. American Thoracic Society, CDC, Infectious Diseases Society of America. Treatment of tuberculosis. *Morbidity and Mortality Weekly Report: Recommendations and Reports*, 2003,52(RR-11):1–77.
8. Saukkonen JJ et al. An official ATS statement: hepatotoxicity of antituberculosis therapy. *American Journal of Respiratory and Critical Care Medicine*, 2006, 174:935–952.

Co-management of HIV and active TB disease

5.1 Chapter objectives

This chapter describes WHO recommendations for:

— HIV testing and counselling of all patients known or suspected to have TB;
— HIV prevention for TB patients;
— treatment of TB in people living with HIV;
— providing co-trimoxazole preventive therapy to all HIV-positive TB patients;
— when to start antiretroviral therapy (ART) and what antiretroviral agents to use;
— drug susceptibility testing and patient monitoring;
— ensuring comprehensive HIV care and support services.

Implementing these recommendations requires collaboration between TB and HIV/AIDS programmes at all levels (*1*, *2*) and will help to reduce the burden of HIV in people diagnosed with TB. Similarly, collaboration is essential to reduce the burden of TB in people living with HIV. (While outside the scope of this chapter, see: *Three I's for reducing the burden of TB in persons living with HIV*: Intensified case-finding (ICF), Isoniazid preventive therapy (IPT) and TB Infection control (IC) for people living with HIV (*3*).)

People living with HIV are more likely to present with extrapulmonary or sputum smear-negative TB, especially as immunosuppression advances (*4*, *5*). This can result in misdiagnosis or delays in diagnosis and, in turn, higher morbidity and mortality. Implementation of the WHO-recommended algorithms to diagnose pulmonary and extrapulmonary TB in HIV-prevalent settings is therefore crucial (*6*). (The treatment of extrapulmonary TB is discussed in Chapter 8.)

5.2 HIV testing and counselling for *all* patients known or suspected to have TB

Irrespective of epidemic setting, WHO recommends HIV testing for patients of all ages who present with signs or symptoms that suggest tuberculosis (*7*), whether TB is suspected or already confirmed. (See also Standard 14 of the ISTC (*8*).) TB is often the first clinical indication that a person has underlying HIV infection, and TB services can be an extremely important entry point to HIV prevention, care and treatment (*1*). In addition, the HIV status of TB patients makes a difference to their TB treatment. (See section 5.4, which includes the new recommendation for daily intensive-phase dosing of anti-TB drugs for HIV-positive TB patients.)

Detecting HIV infection in a TB patient is also critical for the TB patient's household members: HIV-positive TB patients may have household members who are also living with HIV. Testing and counselling should be recommended for children and other immediate family members of all people living with HIV, in cases where horizontal or vertical transmission may have occurred. Within a family-centred approach to HIV testing, once a family member is identified as having HIV, health workers should encourage and actively facilitate HIV testing for other family members. This could be done, where possible and appropriate, through couples or family testing and counselling services (9).[1] Serodiscordant partnerships (in which one partner is HIV-positive and the other is HIV-negative) provide an important opportunity for prevention of HIV transmission (10, 11).

Household contacts of an infectious TB case are a high priority for TB screening and treatment, especially if they are living with HIV (2, 12, 13), and those who are found to have active TB disease need prompt treatment. Among household contacts, people living with HIV (and children, regardless of their HIV status) who do not have active TB are candidates for isoniazid treatment to prevent the development of active TB (3). (See also Standards 16, 18 and 19 of the ISTC (8).)

WHO recommends "provider-initiated" testing, which means that the health care provider recommends HIV testing and counselling as a standard component of care (7). For patients known or suspected to have TB, provider-initiated HIV testing can be done at the same time the sputum samples or chest radiographs are obtained. This is more efficient, and more likely to result in patients learning their HIV status, than referring them elsewhere for HIV testing and counselling (12).

As in the case of client-initiated HIV testing, informed consent, counselling and confidentiality are essential. WHO recommends that providers use "opt-out" approaches (7), meaning that individuals must specifically decline the HIV test after receiving pretest information if they do not want the test to be performed.

The provision of HIV testing by the same health worker who provides the TB treatment (or the provision of HIV testing in the same facility) has been shown to facilitate HIV testing for TB patients (14, 15). If this is not possible, NTPs should take responsibility for ensuring that any referred individual actually goes for a test.

An HIV testing service using rapid assays offers several programmatic advantages. Rapid assays are easy to use and can be carried out by any health care worker who has received appropriate training. Most rapid HIV test kits can be stored at room temperature (up to 30 °C) and can be used for a single test without compromising the integrity of the remaining part of the test kit. Moreover, the diagnostic performance of high-quality rapid assays is comparable to that of traditional enzyme immunoassays, and the short turnaround time ensures that individuals receive their test results quickly. These rapid assays do not require specialized equipment and can be

---

[1] http://www.who.int/hiv/pub/priority_interventions_web.pdf

performed outside the traditional laboratory setting (7). The visibility of the test (to the person being tested) and its speed increase confidence in results and help to avoid clerical errors.

As with conventional HIV assays, a reactive result from the first, highly sensitive, rapid assay requires confirmation by a second, more specific test, typically another rapid assay. If the second test yields non-reactive or indeterminate results, a third test may be performed; if the result is reactive, follow-up HIV testing should be performed on a specimen collected 4 weeks after the initial test. The follow-up testing would rule out possible seroconversion at the time of the initial test as the cause of discrepant testing results and would reveal most technical or clerical errors. The use of rapid assay should be undertaken only with functional quality assurance in place and conducted according to the country's nationally validated testing algorithm. Appropriate post-test counselling should be ensured, with a strong focus on HIV prevention; this will also help prevent the spread of TB.

For more information, see WHO's *Scaling up HIV testing and counselling services: a toolkit for programme managers* (2005), which is available online at: www.who.int/ hiv/topics/vct/toolkit/en/

5.3 HIV prevention in TB patients

National TB control programmes should develop and implement comprehensive HIV prevention strategies for their patients. Appropriate prevention messages and methods should be provided to patients with confirmed or suspected TB, according to their HIV status and local knowledge of the modes of transmission or assessment of risk (1). Harm-reduction measures for TB patients who are injecting drug users should be provided, either by NTPs or through referral linkages to HIV programmes (2).

5.4 TB treatment in people living with HIV

Among treated TB patients, death rates are higher in HIV-positive than in HIV-negative patients. Case-fatality is higher in people living with HIV with smear-negative pulmonary and extrapulmonary TB, as these patients are generally more immunosuppressed than those with smear-positive TB (6). The case-fatality rate is reduced in patients who receive concurrent ART (see section 5.6 below).

The first priority for HIV-positive TB patients is to initiate TB treatment, followed by co-trimoxazole and ART (16) (see sections 5.5 and 5.6 below). For TB diagnosed in a person already taking ART, see section 5.9.

New TB patients[1] living with HIV should be treated with the regimens given in Tables 3.2 and 3.3. However, the three times weekly intensive phase is no longer an

---

[1] New TB patients are those who have had no prior TB treatment or who have been receiving TB treatment for less than 1 month.

option. This new recommendation is based on a systematic review showing that the incidence of relapse and failure among HIV-positive TB patients who were treated with intermittent TB therapy throughout treatment was 2–3 times higher than that in patients who received a daily intensive phase (17). In addition, a study in India showed that HIV-positive patients with pulmonary TB are at higher risk of acquired rifampicin resistance, when failing a three times weekly short-course intermittent regimen (18).

■ **Recommendation 4.1**

TB patients with known positive HIV status and all TB patients living in HIV-prevalent settings[1] should receive daily TB treatment at least during the intensive phase

(Strong/High grade of evidence)

■ **Recommendation 4.2**

For the continuation phase, the optimal dosing frequency is also daily for these patients

(Strong/High grade of evidence)

■ **Recommendation 4.3**

If a daily continuation phase is not possible for these patients, three times weekly dosing during the continuation phase is an acceptable alternative

(Conditional/High or moderate grade of evidence)

In terms of duration of therapy, some experts recommend prolonging TB treatment in persons living with HIV in certain circumstances (19). A systematic review found lower relapse rates in people living with HIV treated with 8 or more months of rifampicin-containing regimens compared with the current recommendation of 6 months. However, the data quality of the studies included in the review was low, and different durations of TB treatment for HIV-positive and HIV-negative individuals would be operationally difficult in resource-constrained and HIV-prevalent settings (17).

■ **Recommendation 4.4**

It is recommended that TB patients who are living with HIV should receive at least the same duration of TB treatment as HIV-negative TB patients

(Strong/High grade of evidence)

HIV-positive TB patients who have been previously treated for TB should receive the same retreatment regimens as HIV-negative TB patients (see Table 3.5).

---

[1] Countries, subnational administrative units, or selected facilities where the HIV prevalence among adult pregnant women is ≥1% or among TB patients is ≥5%.

Rifampicin induces the activity of hepatic enzymes, leading to sub-therapeutic concentrations of some antiretroviral drugs. This is discussed in section 5.6.1 below.

5.5 Co-trimoxazole preventive therapy

In all HIV-positive TB patients, co-trimoxazole preventive therapy should be initiated as soon as possible and given throughout TB treatment. (See also Standard 15 of the ISTC (8).) Co-trimoxazole preventive therapy substantially reduces mortality in HIV-positive TB patients (16, 20). The exact mode of activity is not clear but co-trimoxazole is known to prevent *Pneumocystis jirovecii* and malaria and is likely to have an impact on a range of bacterial infections in HIV-positive TB patients.

A system for providing co-trimoxazole preventive therapy to all people living with HIV who have active TB should be established by TB and HIV programmes. Continuation after TB treatment is completed should be considered in accordance with national guidelines.

For co-trimoxazole dosages, contraindications, and side-effects and their management, see reference 20.

5.6 Antiretroviral therapy

Antiretroviral therapy improves survival in HIV-positive patients (16). In addition, antiretroviral therapy reduces TB rates by up to 90% at an individual level, by 60% at a population level and it reduces TB recurrence rates by 50% (21–22). ART should be initiated for *all* people living with HIV with active TB disease irrespective of CD4 cell count. TB treatment should be started first, followed by ART as soon as possible and within the first 8 weeks of starting TB treatment (23).

5.6.1 What ART regimens to start?

Standardized, simplified ART regimens are used to support HIV treatment programmes so they can reach as many people living with HIV as possible. For the most up-to-date WHO guidance on ART regimens, reference should be made to www. who.int/hiv/pub/guidelines/en

WHO recommends that the first-line ART regimen contain two nucleoside reverse transcriptase inhibitors (NRTIs) plus one non-nucleoside reverse transcriptase inhibitor (NNRTI). These are efficacious, relatively less expensive, have generic and FDC formulations, do not require a cold chain, and preserve a potent new class of agents (protease inhibitors) for second-line regimens. The preferred NRTI backbone is zidovudine (AZT) or tenofovir disoproxil fumarate (TDF), combined with either lamivudine (3TC) or emtricitabine (FTC). For the NNRTI, WHO recommends either efavirenz (EFV) or nevirapine (NVP) (23).

The recommended first-line ART regimens for TB patients are those that contain efavirenz (EFV), since interactions with anti-TB drugs are minimal. In several cohort studies, ART with standard-dose efavirenz and two nucleosides was well tolerated and highly efficacious in achieving complete viral suppression among patients receiving concomitant rifampicin-based TB treatment (24).

Because of concerns related to teratogenicity, efavirenz should not be used in women of childbearing potential without adequate contraception, nor should it be used for women who are in the first trimester of pregnancy. Alternatives are also needed for patients who are intolerant to efavirenz or are infected with a strain of HIV that is resistant to NNRTIs. For those who are unable to tolerate EFV or who have contraindications to an EFV-based regimen, AZT +3TC + NVP or TDF +3TC or FTC + NVP or a triple NRTI regimen (AZT+3TC+ABC or AZT+3TC+TDF) is recommended; the choice of regimen should be based on available regimens within countries. In countries where rifampicin is available, the lead-in dose of nevirapine is not necessary.

In individuals who need TB treatment and who require an ART regimen containing a boosted protease inhibitor (PI), it is recommended to give a rifabutin-based TB treatment. If rifabutin is not available, the use of rifampicin and a boosted antiretroviral regimen containing lopinavir or saquinavir with additional ritonavir dosing is recommended; this regimen should be closely monitored.

5.6.2 When to start ART?

While the optimal time to start ART in relation to the start of TB therapy is not yet clear, one randomized controlled trial provides some evidence for early initiation of antiretroviral therapy in terms of reduced all-cause mortality, improved TB outcomes and reduced incidence of immune reconstitution inflammatory syndrome (IRIS) (25). The recommendations of WHO in 2009 are that TB treatment should be commenced first and ART subsequently commenced, as soon as possible and within the first 8 weeks of starting TB treatment. In this rapidly evolving field, updated information and guidance on antiretroviral therapy is provided by WHO (see: http://www.who.int/hiv/pub guidelines/en).

The rationale for starting ART soon after TB diagnosis is that case-fatality among HIV-TB patients occurs mainly in the first 2 months of TB treatment (16). However, early initiation of ART (within a few weeks of starting TB treatment) means a large number of tablets to ingest, which may discourage treatment adherence; there may also be complications – adverse effects, drug–drug interactions and IRIS.

Mild to moderate IRIS is relatively common in patients with TB started on ART: it has been reported in up to one-third of patients in some studies. However, it is relatively rare in its severe forms (24, 26). The syndrome can present as fever, enlarging lymph nodes, worsening pulmonary infiltrates, or exacerbation of inflammatory changes at other sites. It generally presents within 3 months of the start of ART and is more common when CD4 cell count is low (<50 cells/mm^3). Most cases resolve without intervention and ART can be safely continued (24).

IRIS is a diagnosis of exclusion. Patients with advanced AIDS may show clinical deterioration for a number of other reasons. New opportunistic infections or previously subclinical infections may be unmasked following immune reconstitution and cause clinical worsening. IRIS can also be confused with TB treatment failure. In addition, HIV-positive TB patients may be demonstrating progression of TB disease due to TB drug-resistance. IRIS is not a reason to switch patients to second-line ART, although the ART treatment regimen may need to be adjusted to ensure compatibility with the TB treatment (6).

5.7 Drug susceptibility testing

High mortality rates have been reported among people living with HIV who have drug resistant-TB (26), and rates can exceed 90% in patients coinfected with extensively drug-resistant TB (XDR-TB) and HIV (27, 28). Prompt initiation of appropriate TB treatment (and subsequent initiation of ART) can reduce mortality among people living with HIV who have drug-resistant TB (28).

WHO recommends that NTPs undertake DST at the start of TB therapy in all HIV-positive TB patients, to avoid mortality due to unrecognized drug-resistant TB (25), and strongly encourages the use of rapid DST in sputum smear-positive persons living with HIV (26).

If the country is introducing DST, but does not yet have the resources to test all HIV-positive TB patients, initial NTP policy should be to target DST at the start of TB treatment for patients with previously treated TB, who are very likely to be multidrug-resistant (see section 3.8.1). This group includes patients whose prior TB treatment has failed, who have relapsed or who are returning from default. NTP managers may also chose to target DST for those HIV-positive TB patients with lower CD4 counts (e.g. less than 200 cells/mm^3) given their very high risk of death due to unrecognized drug-resistant TB (26).

5.8 Patient monitoring during TB treatment

(See also Chapter 4.)

Adverse drug effects are common in HIV-positive TB patients, and some toxicities are common to both ART and TB drugs (16). Overlapping toxicities between ART, TB therapy and co-trimoxazole include rash (and, more rarely, hepatic dysfunction), and vigilant monitoring of side-effects is therefore essential (20, 26).

5.9 Considerations when TB is diagnosed in people living with HIV who are already receiving antiretroviral therapy

When TB is diagnosed in patients already receiving ART, TB treatment should be started immediately. There are two issues to consider in such cases: whether ART needs to be modified because of drug–drug interactions or to reduce the potential for overlapping toxicities, and whether the presentation of active TB in a patient on ART constitutes ART failure that requires a change in the ART regimen. Diagnosis and management of ART failure are covered in another WHO document (*29*).

5.10 HIV-related prevention, treatment, care and support

The recommended package of HIV-related prevention, treatment, care and support services and support for people living with HIV should be provided either by TB programmes or by referral to HIV/AIDS programmes (*12, 16*). To improve treatment success, the special needs of particular groups (e.g. drug users, prisoners, migrant populations, other marginalized groups) should be assessed and addressed; their care should be integrated with other services.

A comprehensive AIDS care strategy includes clinical management (prophylaxis, early diagnosis, treatment and follow-up care for opportunistic infections), nursing care (including hygiene promotion and nutritional support), palliative care, home care (including education for care providers and patients' relatives, promoting universal precautions), counselling and social support (*1, 9*). This package of care includes a core set of effective interventions, listed below, that are simple and relatively inexpensive, can improve the quality of life, prevent further transmission of HIV and, in some cases, delay progression of HIV disease and prevent mortality. In addition to ART, these interventions promote health, reduce the risk of HIV transmission to others, and address diseases that most impact the quality and duration of life of adults and adolescents with HIV (*3*):

— reducing the burden of TB via intensified TB case-finding, infection control, and isoniazid preventive therapy;
— psychosocial counselling and support;
— disclosure of HIV status, partner notification and testing and counselling;
— co-trimoxazole prophylaxis;
— preventing fungal infections;
— preventing sexually transmitted and other reproductive tract infections;
— preventing malaria;
— providing selected vaccines (hepatitis B, pneumococcal, influenza, and yellow fever);
— nutrition;
— family planning;
— preventing mother-to-child transmission of HIV;
— needle/syringe programmes and opioid substitution therapy; and water, sanitation and hygiene.

References

1. *Interim policy on collaborative TB/HIV activities.* Geneva, World Health Organization, 2004 (WHO/HTM/TB/2004.330, WHO/HTM/HIV/2004.1).

2. *Implementing the WHO Stop TB strategy: a handbook for national tuberculosis control programmes.* Geneva, World Health Organization, 2008 (WHO/HTM/TB/2008.401).

3. *WHO Three I's Meeting: Intensified case finding (ICF), Isoniazid preventive therapy (IPT) and TB Infection control (IC) for people living with HIV.* Report of a joint World Health Organization HIV/AIDS and TB department meeting. Geneva, World Health Organization, 2008 (available at: http://www.who.int/hiv/pub/meetingreports/WHO_3Is_meeting_report.pdf).

4. *TB/HIV: a clinical manual,* 2nd ed. Geneva, World Health Organization, 2004 (WHO/HTM/TB/2004.329).

5. Getahun H et al. Diagnosis of smear-negative pulmonary tuberculosis in people with HIV infection or AIDS in resource-constrained settings: informing urgent policy changes. *Lancet,* 2007, 369:2042–2049.

6. *Improving the diagnosis and treatment of smear-negative pulmonary and extrapulmonary tuberculosis among adults and adolescents: recommendations for HIV-prevalent and resource-constrained settings.* Geneva, World Health Organization, 2007 (WHO/HTM/TB/2007.379; WHO/HIV/2007.1).

7. WHO, UNAIDS. *Guidance on provider-initiated HIV testing and counselling in health facilities.* Geneva, World Health Organization, 2007.

8. *International Standards for Tuberculosis Care (ISTC),* 2nd ed. The Hague, Tuberculosis Coalition for Technical Assistance, 2009.

9. *Towards universal access: priority interventions for HIV.* Geneva, World Health Organization, 2008.

10. Dunkle KL et al. New heterosexually transmitted HIV infections in married or cohabiting couples in urban Zambia and Rwanda: an analysis of survey and clinical data. *Lancet,* 2008, 371:2183–2191.

11. *Opening up the HIV/AIDS epidemic: guidance on encouraging beneficial disclosure, ethical partner counselling & appropriate use of HIV case-reporting.* Geneva, United Nations Joint Programme on HIV/AIDS, 2000 (available at: http://www.who.int/ethics/topics/opening_up_ethics_and_disclosure_en_2000.pdf).

12. *Tuberculosis care with TB-HIV co-management: integrated management of adolescent and adult illness (IMAI).* Geneva, World Health Organization, 2007.

13. Havlir DV et al. Opportunities and challenges for HIV care in overlapping HIV and TB epidemics. *Journal of the American Medical Association,* 2008, 300:423–430.

14. Nunn P, De Cock K. Measuring progress towards integrated TB-HIV treatment and care services: are countries doing what needs to be done? *International Journal of Tuberculosis and Lung Disease,* 2008, 12(3 Suppl. 1):1.

15. Gasana M et al. Integrating tuberculosis and HIV care in rural Rwanda. *International Journal of Tuberculosis and Lung Disease,* 2008, 12(3 Suppl. 1):39–43.

16. Harries AD, Zachariah R, Lawn SD. Providing HIV care for co-infected tuberculosis patients: a perspective from sub-Saharan Africa. *International Journal of Tuberculosis and Lung Disease,* 2009, 13:6–16.

17. Khan FA et al. Treatment of active tuberculosis in HIV co-infected patients: a systematic review and meta-analysis. *Clinical Infectious Diseases*, 2010 (in press).

18. Swaminathan S et al. *Acquired rifampicin resistance in HIV-infected and uninfected patients with tuberculosis treated with a thrice-weekly short-course regimen*. Poster presented at Conference on Retroviruses and Opportunistic Infections (CROI), Montreal, 2009 (available at: http://www.retroconference.org/2009/Abstracts/35234. htm).

19. American Thoracic Society, CDC, Infectious Diseases Society of America. Treatment of tuberculosis. *Morbidity and Mortality Weekly Report: Recommendations and Reports*, 2003, 52(RR-11):1–77.

20. *Guidelines on co-trimoxazole prophylaxis for HIV-related infections among children, adolescents and adults in resource-limited settings: recommendations for a public health approach*. Geneva, World Health Organization, 2006.

21. Lawn SD, Churchyard G. Epidemiology of HIV-associated tuberculosis. *Current Opinion in HIV and AIDS*, 2009, 4:325–333.

22. Golub JE et al. Long-term effectiveness of diagnosing and treating latent tuberculosis infection in a cohort of HIV-infected and at risk injection drug users. *Journal of Acquired Immune Deficiency Syndromes*, 2008, 49(5):532–537.

23. *Rapid advice for antiretroviral therapy for HIV infection in adults and adolescents*. Geneva, World Health Organization, 2009 (available at http://www.who.int/hiv/pub/ arv/rapid_advice_art.pdf).

24. *Managing drug interactions in the treatment of HIV-related tuberculosis*. Atlanta, GA, Centers for Disease Control and Prevention, 2007 (available at: www.cdc.gov/tb/pub-lications/guidelines/TB_HIV_Drugs/PDF/tbhiv.pdf).

25. Karim SA et al. Initiating ART during TB treatment significantly increases survival: results of a randomized controlled clinical trial in TB/HIV-co-infected patients in South Africa. Paper presented at Conference on Retroviruses and Opportunistic Infections (CROI), Montreal, 2009 (available at: http://www.retroconference.org/2009/ Abstracts/34255.htm).

26. *Guidelines for the programmatic management of drug-resistant tuberculosis: emergency update 2008*. Geneva, World Health Organization, 2008 (WHO/HTM/TB/ 2008.402).

27. Gandhi NR et al. Extensively drug-resistant tuberculosis as a cause of death in patients co-infected with tuberculosis and HIV in a rural area of South Africa. *Lancet*, 2006, 368:1575–1580.

28. Wells CD et al. HIV infection and multidrug-resistant tuberculosis: the perfect storm. *Journal of Infectious Diseases*, 2007, 196(Suppl. 1):S86–S107.

29. *Essential prevention and care interventions for adults and adolescents living with HIV in resource-limited settings*. Geneva, World Health Organization, 2008.

6

Supervision and patient support

6.1 Chapter objectives

This chapter describes:

— the role of the patient, the TB programme, other providers, and the community in the cure of TB;
— treatment supervision and directly observed therapy;
— patient-centred care;
— measures to prevent interruption of treatment.

Adherence to TB treatment is crucial to achieving cure while avoiding the emergence of drug resistance. Regular and complete medication intake gives individual TB patients the best chance of cure and also protects the community from the spread of TB. The emergence and spread of MDR- and XDR-TB further reinforces the absolute necessity of helping a TB patient to not miss any drug doses. In the Stop TB Strategy, supervision and patient support remain the cornerstone of DOTS and help programmes to achieve the treatment success target of 85% (1).

6.2 Roles of the patient, TB programme staff, the community and other providers

Cure can be achieved only if the patient and the health service staff work together (2). Other health care providers and the community also have important roles to play.

6.2.1 Patient as partner

According to the Patients' Charter for TB Care, patients are not passive recipients of services but active partners (3). They have the right to care, dignity, information, privacy, food supplements and/or other types of support and incentives, if needed. They also have the right to participate in TB programme development, implementation and evaluation. Patients have the responsibility of sharing information with the health provider, following treatment, contributing to community health, and showing solidarity by passing expertise gained during treatment to others in the community. Because of their first-hand TB experience, their involvement in stigma-reduction activities in the community and supporting treatment completion of other patients can be highly effective.

6.2.2 Role of the NTP and its staff

Because TB is a public health problem and its transmission poses a risk to the community, ensuring regular intake of all the drugs by the patient is a responsibility of the health staff and of the NTP. To facilitate patient adherence, NTPs need to establish and maintain systems that maximize patient access to care, and train and supervise health workers to provide patient-centred care. Factors such as the type of drug regimen (daily or intermittent), the type of drug formulation (fixed-dose combinations or separate drugs) as well as the circumstances and characteristics of the patient should be considered in organizing patient supervision (see section 6.4).

To support patient adherence, it is critical for the NTP to implement two additional components of the Stop TB Strategy: engaging other care providers and involving communities (1).

6.2.3 Engaging providers outside the TB programme

WHO has developed guidance on engaging all health care providers to take on TB tasks according to their capacity (4). For example, public and private practitioners can successfully provide DOTS in collaboration with the NTP. At a minimum, any practitioner treating a patient for TB must be capable of (5):

— discussing the condition and the treatment being given to the patient;
— recognizing and managing adverse effects of medications, and making referrals if necessary;
— assessing the patient's adherence to the regimen and addressing poor adherence when it occurs (ISTC Standard 7 (6));
— completing the appropriate documentation;
— collaborating with the local public health services;
— ensuring that the patient accepts the proposed care.

6.2.4 Community involvement

Another component of the Stop TB Strategy is to empower communities (1). Community involvement refers to partnership and shared responsibility with health services (7). Social mobilization can create demand for quality-assured TB services and help the community to avail itself of these services.

In community-based care, a TB treatment supporter shares with the TB patient responsibility for the successful completion of treatment; he or she provides therapy under supervision as well as social and psychological support (8). Community-based care can help to expand access to care but requires a strong reporting system, access to laboratory facilities, and a secure drug supply. Treatment supporters need regular contact with NTP staff to ensure that motivation and successful outcomes are maintained. Community based TB care is a sign of commitment by the NTP to partnership with the community.

6.3 Supervised treatment

Supervised treatment refers to helping patients to take their TB medications regularly and to complete TB treatment. It is also meant to ensure that the providers give proper care and are able to detect treatment interruption. One example of treatment supervision is recording each dose of anti-TB drugs on the patient's treatment card.

Directly observed therapy (DOT), a recommended method of supervision, should be seen as a part of a support package that addresses patients' needs. This package should help to ensure that DOT is sensitive to, and supportive of, the patient's needs. A treatment supporter observing intake of every dose ensures that a TB patient takes the right anti-TB drugs, in the right doses, at the right intervals. Regular supervision and support help to maintain frequent communication between the patient and a health worker or treatment observer; this provides more opportunities for TB education, identification and resolution of obstacles to treatment, and early identification of non-adherence – allowing interventions to return the patient to the prescribed treatment. Regular supervision also allows the prompt detection and management of adverse drug reactions and clinical worsening of TB.

As a method of supervision recommended by WHO, DOT has been the subject of much debate (9). A systematic review of six controlled trials comparing DOT with self-administered therapy concluded that DOT did not improve outcomes (10). However, this review took no account of the patient support services provided in addition to the routine "supervised swallowing" or of the impact of DOT in preventing the emergence of drug resistance (11). Other reviews found DOT to be associated with high cure and treatment completion rates (9, 12). The highest success rates were achieved in programmes that used DOT in the context of a full support package, with components such as incentives and enablers (discussed in section 6.4 below) (13, 14).

Direct observation of each dose of drugs is most critical in the intensive phase, when intermittent dosing is used during either phase, and in the treatment of, for example, psychologically handicapped patients, prison inmates, or patients receiving second-line anti-TB drugs. Supervised treatment should be carried out in a context-specific and patient-friendly manner. There must be flexibility in how DOT is applied, with adaptation to different settings that are convenient to the patient. The whole purpose of treatment observation would be defeated if it were to limit access to care, turn patients away from treatment, or add to their hardships.

Depending on the local conditions, supervision may be undertaken at a health facility, in the workplace, in the community or at home. A treatment supporter must be identified for each TB patient; he or she should be a person acceptable to, and chosen with, the patient. For TB patients who live close to a health facility, the treatment supporter will be one of the staff in the health facility, and this is the ideal choice if convenient to the patient. Collaboration with other programmes allows the identification of staff from these programmes who may observe TB treatment.

For TB patients who live far away from a health facility the treatment observer will be a community health worker or a trained and supervised local community member. With suitable training and monitoring, HIV/AIDS community care providers can observe TB treatment. Cured TB patients may be successful DOT providers, as can traditional healers, friends, co-workers, family members, neighbours, religious leaders, etc. (*15*); in fact, any willing person who is acceptable to the patient and answerable to the health system can be a treatment supporter.

The NTP is responsible for training and monitoring the non-medical treatment observers. There must be a clearly defined line of accountability from NTP staff to general health services staff and the treatment supporter. It is important to ensure confidentiality and the acceptability of supervised treatment to the patient. The drugs should remain with the treatment supporter and be given to the patient only at the time of ingestion.

There may be an incentive for community members to become observers of TB treatment. Incentives for volunteers and patients may be considered, bearing in mind the advantages and disadvantages of incentive schemes (*16*).

Detailed instructions for informing the patient and family about TB and its treatment and for arranging supervised treatment (including identifying and preparing a community TB treatment supporter) are contained in WHO's training modules for health facility staff (*17*).

6.4 Using a patient-centred approach to care and treatment delivery

Many NTPs now have considerable experience in implementing adherence promotion strategies that work and in tailoring DOT to a given context. Locally appropriate measures should be taken to identify and address physical, financial, social and cultural (as well as health system) obstacles to accessing TB treatment services (*18*). Particular attention should be paid to the poorest and most vulnerable groups. Also useful are explicit efforts to address gender issues, improve staff attitudes, and enhance communication. It is essential that these approaches be based on ethical principles regarding the needs, rights, capabilities and responsibilities of patients, their families and their communities. (See also Standards 7, 9 and 17 of the ISTC (*6*).)

For any chosen method of supervision and administration of treatment, a programme must show high sputum smear conversion and cure rates, under routine conditions, in both rural and urban areas. If evaluation shows suboptimal results, the method of supervision and administration of the regimen should be altered and tested in demonstration and training districts.

In addition to supervised treatment (or DOT), measures to support patient adherence to regular and complete treatment include:

- A regular supply of drugs
  — provided free of charge;
  — allocated in patient kits, to ensure that drugs for the full course of treatment are reserved for the patient at the outset of treatment;
  — in fixed-dose combinations and blister packs, to help reduce medication error as well as facilitating adherence.

- Accessible, high-quality, continuous ambulatory TB care (if treatment is health facility-based)
  — expanding treatment outlets in the poorest rural and urban settings and involving providers who practise close to where patients live (thus reducing travel costs and loss of time and wages);
  — convenient clinic hours with minimal waiting times;
  — adequate numbers of motivated health workers with managerial support;
  — flexibility to make appropriate arrangements for transfer to another facility (*19*);
  — ability to make arrangements upon release from prison or hospital to continue care on an ambulatory basis in the patient's community.

- Positive action to remove barriers to treatment and care
  — ensuring that all services provided are affordable (if not free), and eliminating cost of care;
  — appropriate patient education, including information regarding the regimen, duration and possible treatment outcomes, provided repeatedly by well-trained and considerate staff;
  — prompt detection and management of adverse drug reactions;
  — availability of other forms of treatment support (such as community, workplace, or other) are available when facility-based treatment poses an obstacle for the patient;
  — provision or financing of transportation, and other treatment enablers that can compensate patients for the indirect costs of care;
  — provision of incentives such as food or hygienic packages for patients and their families, if appropriate for the context and for the patient;
  — patient and peer support groups, which may help also reduce stigma;
  — referrals for psychological, social and legal support and other services including substance abuse treatment; joint (integrated) support for TB patients with addictive behaviours;
  — ready availability of concomitant HIV treatment.

- Availability of hospitalization

Hospitalization is essential for severely ill patients and for those with complications or associated conditions requiring closer clinical monitoring. It might also be an alternative, especially during the initial phase of treatment, for a small number of patients for whom other means of ensuring treatment adherence and support are not available. However, hospitalization per se does not ensure regular drug intake or completion of the treatment. Patient-centred support and supervision are just as important to success in an inpatient setting as in the community.

6.5 Prevention of treatment interruption

Globally, 5% of new smear-positive cases treated under DOTS in 2006 defaulted, but this ranges from <1% to 13% in the world's 22 high-burden countries. Default includes patients who have interrupted treatment but also patients who have died or transferred out and whose outcomes are unknown to the NTP treatment staff. The true status of the "defaulting patient" must be ascertained: if defaulting is due to treatment interruption, and if it could be prevented, additional countries would be able to achieve the global TB control target of 85% treatment success. Treatment interruption can be prevented – or limited so that a patient does not default entirely from therapy (20). Promoting adherence through a patient-centred approach is probably more effective in preventing treatment interruption than devoting resources to tracing patients who default.

Among the major factors that influence treatment interruption are comorbid conditions such as substance abuse or mental illness, access to treatment (distance, cost of transport) (21), time and wages lost, quality and speed of drug delivery, extent of knowledge about TB and the need to complete treatment, and flexibility for transfer to another facility.

As described in section 6.4, supervised treatment can help prevent interruptions. When patients self-administer treatment, they often take drugs irregularly, and tracing is difficult and often unproductive; there is also a much longer delay between interruption of treatment and action by the health system.

Whenever the patient visits the health facility, the need for regular and complete intake of treatment should be reinforced and any problems that may cause interruption should be identified. At registration, sufficient time should be set aside for meeting with the patient (and preferably also the patient's family members or a designated treatment supporter). This initial meeting provides an important opportunity to inform the patient about the duration of treatment. During the meeting, it is vital to record the patient's address and other relevant addresses (e.g. partner or spouse, parents, place of work or study, or private doctor who may be consulted) as well as explain the need to consult ahead of time in case of a change of address. This maximizes the likelihood of locating patients who interrupt treatment. Recording mobile telephone numbers for the patient and family has proved valuable in many settings.

Where resources permit, it is helpful for a health staff member to accompany the patient to his or her residence. This allows verification of the patient's exact address and provides an opportunity to arrange for screening of household contacts, especially children under 5 years of age and those of any age who may have TB symptoms or be living with HIV.

In the meeting with the patient at the end of the initial phase of treatment, the health worker should reassess his or her needs and enquire about plans (work, family, moving to another location) that may affect the continuation phase of treatment (*19*). Any changes in the regimen should be discussed and all concerns should be addressed.

References

1. *The Stop TB Strategy: building on and enhancing DOTS to meet the TB-related Millennium Development Goals.* Geneva, World Health Organization, 2006 (WHO/HTM/TB/2006.368).
2. Williams G et al. Care during the intensive phase: promotion of adherence. *International Journal of Tuberculosis and Lung Disease*, 2008, 12:601–605.
3. *Patients' charter for tuberculosis care: patients' rights and responsibilities.* Geneva, World Care Council, 2006.
4. *Engaging all health care providers in TB control: guidance on implementing public-private mix approaches.* Geneva, World Health Organization, 2006 (WHO/HTM/TB/2006.360).
5. *TB guidelines for nurses in the care and control of tuberculosis and multi-drug resistant tuberculosis.* Geneva, International Council of Nurses, 2008.
6. *International Standards for Tuberculosis Care (ISTC)*, 2nd ed. The Hague, Tuberculosis Coalition for Technical Assistance, 2009.
7. *Community involvement in tuberculosis care and prevention. Towards partnerships for health: guiding principles and recommendations based on a WHO review.* Geneva, World Health Organization, 2008 (WHO/HTM/TB/2008.397).
8. Raviglione M, ed. *Reichman and Hershfield's tuberculosis: a comprehensive, international approach*, 3rd ed. New York, Informa Healthcare, 2006.
9. Frieden TR, Sbarbaro JA. Promoting adherence to treatment for tuberculosis: the importance of direct observation. *Bulletin of the World Health Organization*, 2007, 85:407–409.
10. Volmink J, Garner P. Directly observed therapy for treating tuberculosis. *Cochrane Database of Systematic Reviews*, 2007, (4)(4):CD003343.
11. Rusen ID et al. Cochrane systematic review of directly observed therapy for treating tuberculosis: good analysis of the wrong outcome. *International Journal of Tuberculosis and Lung Disease*, 2007, 11:120–121.
12. Hopewell PC et al. International standards for tuberculosis care. *Lancet Infectious Diseases*, 2006, 6:710–725.
13. Suarez PG et al. The dynamics of tuberculosis in response to 10 years of intensive control effort in Peru. *Journal of Infectious Diseases*, 2001, 184:473–478.
14. Chaulk CP, Kazandjian VA. Directly observed therapy for treatment completion of pulmonary tuberculosis: consensus statement of the public health tuberculosis guidelines panel. *Journal of the American Medical Association*, 1998, 279:943–948.
15. Pungrassami P et al. Practice of directly observed treatment (DOT) for tuberculosis in southern Thailand: comparison between different types of DOT observers. *International Journal of Tuberculosis and Lung Disease*, 2002, 6:389–395.

16. Beith A, Eichler R, Weil D. Performance-based incentives for health: a way to improve tuberculosis detection and treatment completion? Washington, DC, Center for Global Development, 2007 (CGD Working Paper, no. 122).

17. *Management of tuberculosis: training for health facility staff.* Geneva, World Health Organization, 2003 (WHO/CDS/TB/2003.314).

18. Munro SA et al. Patient adherence to tuberculosis treatment: a systematic review of qualitative research. *PLoS Medicine*, 2007, 4:e238.

19. Williams G et al. Care during the continuation phase. *International Journal of Tuberculosis and Lung Disease*, 2008, 2:731–735.

20. Williams G et al. *Best practice of the care for patients with tuberculosis: a guide for low income countries.* Paris, International Union Against Tuberculosis and Lung Disease, 2007.

21. Shargie EB, Lindtjorn B. Determinants of treatment adherence among smear-positive pulmonary tuberculosis patients in southern Ethiopia. *PLoS Medicine*, 2007, 4:e37.

Treatment of drug–resistant tuberculosis

7.1 Chapter objectives

This chapter describes:

— the Green Light Committee – one of the sources of support to countries establishing a drug-resistant TB component and integrating it into their NTP;

— groups of drugs used to treat MDR-TB, and the principles for constructing an MDR-TB regimen;

— programmatic strategies for MDR-TB treatment – how to select the standard MDR-TB regimen (and considerations for an individualized approach once DST results are available);

— how to monitor MDR-TB patients, determine when to stop the injectable agent, and decide when treatment is completed;

— how to treat TB with resistance patterns other than MDR;

— recording and reporting of drug-resistant TB cases.

This chapter highlights key concepts for treating drug-resistant TB – preventing the development of drug resistance, and detecting it promptly when it does occur, are discussed in Chapters 3 to 6.

This chapter is intended to serve as a brief overview. Managers of NTPs who are establishing a drug-resistant component and integrating it into their programmes are strongly urged to seek expert consultation (see section 7.2 below) and to review the 2008 or subsequent editions of the WHO *Guidelines for the programmatic management of drug resistant TB (1)*.[1] (See also Standard 12 of the ISTC (2).)

7.2 Green Light Committee Initiative

In designing the country's MDR-TB treatment component and integrating it into the national programme, NTP managers are strongly encouraged to make full use of the Green Light Committee (GLC; www.who.int/tb/challenges/mdr/greenlightcommittee). The GLC is a subgroup of the MDR-TB Working Group of the Stop TB Partnership, and an advisory body of WHO that promotes access to (and monitors the use of) quality-assured, life-saving MDR-TB treatment.

---

[1] That publication also provides in-depth guidance on the many facets of MDR-TB management, including management of side-effects and indications for surgery.

Through the GLC Initiative, NTPs have access to:

— expertise in programmatic management of drug-resistant TB based on best available evidence and collective experience;
— high-quality drugs to treat drug-resistant TB at concessional prices;
— support through a wide network of technical partners;
— peer support and knowledge-sharing with other GLC-approved programmes;
— independent external monitoring and evaluation.

7.3 Groups of drugs to treat MDR-TB

For MDR treatment, anti-TB drugs are grouped according to efficacy, experience of use and drug class (Table 7.1). All the first-line anti-TB drugs are in Group 1, except streptomycin, which is classified with the other injectable agents in Group 2. All the drugs in Groups 2–5 (except streptomycin) are second-line, or reserve, drugs. The features of the drugs within each group, including cross-resistance, are discussed in more detail below. Cross-resistance means that resistance mutations (in *M. tuberculosis* bacteria) to one anti-TB drug may confer resistance to some or all of the members of the drug family and, less commonly, to members of different drug families (*1*).

Group 1. Group 1 drugs are the most potent and best tolerated. If there is good laboratory evidence and clinical history that suggests that a drug from this group is effective, it should be used. If a Group 1 drug was used in a previous regimen that failed, its efficacy should be questioned even if the DST result suggests susceptibility. The newer rifamycins, such as rifabutin, have very high rates of cross-resistance to rifampicin.

Group 2. All patients should receive a Group 2 injectable agent if susceptibility is documented or suspected. Among aminoglycosides, kanamycin or amikacin is the first choice of an injectable agent, given the high rates of streptomycin resistance in drug-resistant TB. In addition, both these agents are inexpensive, cause less otoxicity than streptomycin, and have been used extensively for the treatment of drug-resistant TB. Amikacin and kanamycin are considered to be very similar and have a high frequency of cross-resistance. If an isolate is resistant to both streptomycin and kanamycin, or if DRS data show high rates of resistance to amikacin and kanamycin, capreomycin (a polypeptide) should be used.

Group 3. All patients should receive a Group 3 medication if the *M. tuberculosis* strain is susceptible or if the agent is thought to have efficacy. One of the higher generation fluoroquinolones, such as levofloxacin or moxifloxacin, is the fluoroquinolone of choice. Ciprofloxacin is no longer recommended to treat drug-susceptible or drug-resistant TB.

Group 4. Ethionamide (or protionamide) is often added to the treatment regimen because of its low cost. If cost is not a constraint, *p*-aminosalicylic acid (PAS) may be added first, given that the enteric-coated formulas are relatively well tolerated and that

Table 7.1   GROUPS OF DRUGS TO TREAT MDR-TB[a]

Group	Drugs (abbreviations)
Group 1: First-line oral agents	• pyrazinamide (Z) • ethambutol (E) • rifabutin (Rfb)
Group 2: Injectable agents	• kanamycin (Km) • amikacin (Am) • capreomycin (Cm) • streptomycin (S)
Group 3: Fluoroquinolones	• levofloxacin (Lfx) • moxifloxacin (Mfx) • ofloxacin (Ofx)
Group 4: Oral bacteriostatic second-line agents	• para-aminosalicylic acid (PAS) • cycloserine (Cs) • terizidone (Trd) • ethionamide (Eto) • protionamide (Pto)
Group 5: Agents with unclear role in treatment of drug resistant-TB	• clofazimine (Cfz) • linezolid (Lzd) • amoxicillin/clavulanate (Amx/Clv) • thioacetazone (Thz) • imipenem/cilastatin (Ipm/Cln) • high-dose isoniazid (high-dose H)[b] • clarithromycin (Clr)

[a] Adapted from Table 7.1 and Figure 7.2 of reference *1*.
[b] High-dose isoniazid is defined as 16–20 mg/kg/day. Some experts recommend using high-dose isoniazid in the presence of resistance to low concentrations of isoniazid (>1% of bacilli resistant to 0.2 µg/ml but susceptible to 1 µg/ml of isoniazid), whereas isoniazid is not recommended for high-dose resistance (>1% of bacilli resistant to 1 µg/ml of isoniazid) (*1*).

there is no cross-resistance to other agents. When two agents are needed, cycloserine can be added. Since the combination of ethionamide (or protionamide) and PAS often causes a high incidence of gastrointestinal side-effects and hypothyroidism, these agents are usually used together only when three Group 4 agents are needed: ethionamide (or protionamide), cycloserine and PAS. Terizidone can be used instead of cycloserine and is assumed to be equally efficacious.

Group 5. Group 5 drugs are not recommended by WHO for routine use in drug-resistant TB treatment because their contribution to the efficacy of multidrug regimens is unclear. They can be used in cases where it is impossible to design adequate regimens with the medicines from Groups 1–4, such as in patients with XDR-TB. They should be used in consultation with an expert in the treatment of drug-resistant TB.

7.4 General principles in designing an MDR-TB treatment regimen

The general principles in Table 7.2 apply whether an NTP manager is selecting an empirical or standard MDR-TB regimen for the country[1] or a clinician is constructing a regimen for an individual patient. These principles also apply to XDR-TB cases. (Individual patient-specific information, which is part of the clinician's evaluation of each patient before starting the MDR regimen, is given in parentheses in the table.)

Treatment regimens should consist of at least four drugs with either certain, or almost certain, effectiveness. Where evidence about the effectiveness of a certain drug is unclear, the drug can be part of the regimen but it should not be depended upon for success. Often, more than four drugs may be started if the susceptibility pattern is unknown or the effectiveness of one or more agents is questionable.

Susceptibility testing for isoniazid, rifampicin, the fluoroquinolones, and the injectable agents is fairly reliable. For other agents it is less reliable, and basing individualized treatments on DST for these agents should be avoided. The clinical effectiveness or ineffectiveness of a drug cannot be predicted by DST with 100% certainty.

Each dose in an MDR regimen is given as DOT throughout the treatment. See reference *1* for detailed information on each drug, including adverse effects, contraindications, monitoring, and dosing based on weight bands.

7.5 Programmatic strategies for treatment of MDR-TB

Programmatic approaches to MDR-TB treatment depend in part on the type of laboratory method used to confirm MDR (see Figure 7.1). Once MDR-TB is confirmed (by either type of laboratory method), patients can be treated with:

— a standard MDR regimen (standardized approach); or
— an individually tailored regimen, based on DST of additional drugs.

For NTPs using conventional DST methods, there is often a delay of months before results are available to confirm or exclude MDR. These countries need to consider MDR treatment at two stages: when MDR is suspected but laboratory confirmation is pending, and once MDR is confirmed. While awaiting results, patients who are highly likely to have MDR-TB (such as those whose prior treatment has failed) need an empirical MDR regimen. If MDR is confirmed, this regimen may be continued, or it may be tailored on the basis of susceptibility to drugs other than isoniazid and rifampicin, as discussed in section 7.7.

NTPs using rapid molecular-based DST will be able to confirm MDR-TB within 1–2 days,[2] and then can initiate treatment with a standard MDR regimen immediately, or

---

[1] Programmatic strategies for MDR-TB treatment (standardized or individualized approaches) are described in section 7.5.
[2] Line probe assays detect resistance to rifampicin alone or in combination with isoniazid resistance. Overall high accuracy for detection of MDR is retained when rifampicin resistance alone is used as a marker for MDR (*3, 4*).

Table 7.2 GENERAL PRINCIPLES FOR DESIGNING MDR-TB TREATMENT REGIMENS[a]

Principles	Comments
1. Use at least 4 drugs certain to be effective	The more of the following factors are present, the more likely it is that the drug will be effective: • Resistance to these drugs is known from surveys to be rare in similar patients. • DST results show susceptibility to drugs for which there is good laboratory reliability: injectable agents and fluoroquinolones. • The drug is not commonly used in the area. • (For decisions about an individual patient – no prior history of treatment failure with the drug; no known close contacts with resistance to the drug.)
2. Do not use drugs for which there is the possibility of cross-resistance	• Many antituberculosis agents exhibit cross-resistance both within and across drug classes (see section 7.3).
3. Eliminate drugs that are not safe	• Quality of the drug is unknown. • (For decisions about an individual patient – known severe allergy or unmanageable intolerance; high risk of severe adverse drug effects such as renal failure, deafness, hepatitis, depression and/or psychosis.)
4. Include drugs from Groups 1–5 in a hierarchical order based on potency (see Table 7.1 and section 7.3)	• Use any of the first-line oral agents (Group 1) that are likely to be effective. • Use an effective aminoglycoside or polypeptide by injection (Group 2).[b] • Use a fluoroquinolone (Group 3). • Use the remaining Group 4 drugs to complete a regimen of at least four effective drugs. • For regimens with fewer than four effective drugs, consider adding two Group 5 drugs. The total number of drugs will depend on the degree of uncertainty, and regimens often contain five to seven.

[a] Adapted from Table 7.3 of reference *1*.
[b] Avoid streptomycin even if DST suggests susceptibility because of high rates of resistance with resistant TB strains and higher incidence of ototoxicity.

may tailor the regimen later when DST results for second-line drugs become available, as discussed in section 7.7.

Standardized and individualized approaches each have advantages. Standard MDR-TB regimens (5) make it easier to estimate drug needs, to order, manage and distribute drug stocks, and to train personnel in the treatment of MDR-TB patients. Even when standard regimens are used throughout treatment, patients experiencing severe adverse effects will need to have their MDR treatment individualized. Thus all programmes need some capacity to individualize treatment.

Changing to an *individualized* regimen (once DST results are available for additional drugs beyond isoniazid and rifampicin) is advantageous because it:

- Allows clinicians to design a regimen with knowledge of resistance to particular injectables and fluoroquinolones, which is especially important if patients have received second-line drugs in the past. This knowledge helps in avoiding the use of toxic and expensive drugs to which the patient's *M. tuberculosis* is found to be resistant.

- Allows clinicians to tailor the regimen in settings with high rates of resistance to second-line drugs where it may be difficult to find a standard regimen that is appropriate for all patients.

- Provides flexibility if patients experience adverse effects related to one drug.

In some settings, individualized regimens may achieve higher cure rates than standard MDR regimens (6).

Figure 7.1   DIAGRAM OF MDR TREATMENT STRATEGIES DEPENDING ON LABORATORY METHOD TO CONFIRM MDR

Treatment timeline (time since TB diagnosis)

TB diagnosis ◊-------/--------/-------/-------/-------/-------/-------/-------/-------/-------/----◊

Countries using conventional methods to detect MDR:

While awaiting DST results for isoniazid, rifampicin; MDR-TB is suspected	Once MDR is confirmed
Empirical treatment with MDR regimen	Continue **standard** MDR regimen *or* Change to **individualized** MDR regimen (once susceptibility testing for second-line drugs is available)

Countries using rapid method to detect MDR:

Once MDR is confirmed[a]
Standard MDR regimen *or* **Individualized** MDR regimen (once susceptibility testing for second-line drugs is available)

[a]   Little waiting; takes approximately 1–2 days to detect MDR.

7.6 Selection of the country's standard MDR-TB regimen

A country's standard MDR regimen can be used while confirmation of MDR is awaited (i.e. empirically) or once MDR is confirmed. In selecting the standard MDR regimen, NTP managers are strongly urged to seek expert consultation (see section 7.2 above) and to review planned regimens (1). The discussion below provides a general overview only.

The standard MDR regimen is constructed using the principles outlined in section 7.5 and Table 7.2. To identify the drugs that are likely to be effective, the NTP manager needs to gather information about the level of MDR in the patients to be treated, as well as the pattern of resistance to other Group 1 drugs, injectable agents (Group 2) and fluoroquinolones (Group 3). Ideally, drug resistance data will be available from patients who have similar histories of previous treatment to the patients who will actually be treated. The data should:

— include a large enough number of patients to give confidence in the results;
— be based on reliable laboratory methods for DST;
— accurately describe the patients' treatment history to distinguish between those in whom the first or subsequent treatment failed, those who have relapsed, and those who are returning after defaulting.

As described in section 3.8.2, the NTP manager should access any drug resistance surveys or available surveillance data. If data show very different drug resistance patterns across groups of previously treated patients, there may need to be more than one standard MDR regimen.

The NTP manager also needs to assess the use and quality of anti-TB drugs in the country. The following information, if available, will be helpful:

- Current and past NTP standard regimens for new and previously treated patients.

- History of drug availability and sales in pharmacies. Some second line anti-TB drugs may have been used only rarely and will probably be effective in MDR regimens. Those that have been used extensively are highly likely to be ineffective.

- Quality assurance of drugs used within and outside the NTP.

Box 7.1 provides an example of how to design a standard regimen.

7.7 Selection of individualized MDR-TB regimens

Individually designed regimens are based on the patient's history of past drug use and on DST of isoniazid, rifampicin, the second-line injectable agents and a fluoroquinolone. Every effort should be made to supplement the patient's memory of treatment with objective records from previous health care providers. A detailed clinical history can help suggest which drugs are likely to be ineffective. Although resistance can develop in less than 1 month, if a patient has used a drug for more than 1 month

---

BOX 7.1

EXAMPLE[a]

Survey data from 93 consecutively enrolled relapsed patients from a resource-constrained area show that 11% have MDR-TB. Of these MDR-TB cases, 45% are resistant to ethambutol and 29% are resistant to streptomycin. Resistance to other drugs is unknown; however, there is virtually no use of any of the second-line drugs in the area. What retreatment strategy is recommended in this group of relapse patients?

Given the relatively low rate of MDR-TB in this group, the following strategy is planned:

- All relapse patients will be started on isoniazid, rifampicin, pyrazinamide, ethambutol and streptomycin, i.e. the retreatment regimen using first-line drugs.
- DST of isoniazid and rifampicin will be done at the start of treatment to identify the 11% of MDR-TB patients who will not do well on the retreatment regimen of first-line drugs.
- Those patients identified with MDR-TB will be switched to the standard regimen:
  — 8 months of pyrazinamide, kanamycin, ofloxacin, protionamide, and cycloserine, followed by 12 months of ofloxacin, protionamide, and cycloserine.
  — The regimen contains four drugs rarely used in the area and is also relatively inexpensive.
- A small DST survey is planned to document the prevalence of resistance to the regimen's five drugs in 30 relapse patients found to have MDR-TB. If this survey shows high resistance to any of the proposed drugs, redesign of the regimen will be considered.

Note: The regimen proposed in this answer is only one example of an adequate regimen.

[a] Reproduced from *Guidelines for the programmatic management of drug-resistant tuberculosis: emergency update 2008* (1).

---

with persistently positive smears or cultures, the strain should – as a general rule – be considered as "probably resistant" to that drug, even if DST results indicate that it is susceptible.

DST results should complement, rather than invalidate, other sources of data on the likely effectiveness of a specific drug. For example, if a history of prior anti-TB drug use suggests that a drug is likely to be ineffective, that drug should not be relied on as one of the four core drugs in the regimen, even if DST shows the strain to be susceptible. Alternatively, if the patient has never taken a particular drug and resistance to that drug is extremely uncommon in the community, DST results that indicate resistance may be the result case of a laboratory error or of the limited specificity of DST for some second-line drugs.[1]

---

[1] Since a fluoroquinolone and an injectable agent form the backbone of MDR treatment, they should be used even if the patient's *M. tuberculosis* demonstrates resistance to all available drugs in these two classes (7, 8).

Another important limitation is the turnaround time for DST results: the patient may have already received months of treatment by the time DST results become available from the laboratory. The possibility of further acquired resistance developing during this time must be considered. If there is a high probability of acquired resistance to a particular drug after collection of the specimen for DST, that drug should not be counted as one of the four drugs in the core regimen (but can be included as an adjunctive agent).

7.8 Monitoring the MDR-TB patient

Close monitoring is essential during treatment of MDR-TB patients. To assess treatment response, sputum smears and cultures should be performed monthly until smear and culture conversion. (Conversion is defined as two consecutive negative smears and cultures taken 30 days apart.) After conversion, the minimum frequency recommended for bacteriological monitoring is monthly for smears and quarterly for cultures. Monitoring of MDR-TB patients by a clinician should be at least monthly until sputum conversion, then every 2–3 months. Each patient's weight should be monitored monthly.

Second-line drugs have many more adverse effects than the first-line anti-TB drugs, but management of these adverse effects is possible even in resource-poor settings. At every DOT and clinician encounter, the patient should be screened for side-effects of medication. It is also essential for patients to be aware of possible side-effects and to have access to clinical and laboratory services to help detect side-effects, and medications to treat adverse effects when they occur. For more details on patient monitoring, see reference 1. Timely and intensive monitoring for, and management of, adverse effects caused by second-line drugs are essential for MDR-TB treatment.

7.9 Duration of treatment for MDR-TB

In MDR-TB treatment, the intensive phase is defined by the duration of treatment with the injectable agent. The injectable agent should be continued for a minimum of 6 months, and for at least 4 months after the patient first becomes and remains smear- or culture-negative. Review of the patient's cultures, smears, X-rays and clinical status may also aid in deciding whether or not to continue an injectable agent longer than the above recommendation, particularly in the case of patients for whom the susceptibility pattern is unknown, effectiveness of one or more agents is questionable, or extensive or bilateral pulmonary disease is present.

Culture conversion also determines the overall duration of MDR treatment. These guidelines recommend continuing therapy for a minimum of 18 months after culture conversion. Extension of therapy to 24 months may be indicated in chronic cases with extensive pulmonary damage.

7.10 Treating TB with resistance patterns other than MDR

Cases with drug resistance patterns other than MDR will be detected by DST. The design of regimens for mono- and poly-resistant cases of TB is recommended for programmes with good infrastructure that are capable of treating MDR-TB. Individually designed treatments for mono- and poly-resistance are often determined by a review panel that meets periodically. The panel reviews treatment history, DST patterns and the possibility of strains of *M. tuberculosis* having acquired new resistance, and then determines the regimen. For suggested regimens according to the pattern of drug resistance, see reference *1*.

It is essential to remember that the DST result reflects the bacterial population at the time the sputum was collected and not necessarily the bacterial population in the patient at the time the result is reported. During the interval between collection of the specimen and receipt of the results, the *M. tuberculosis* bacteria may have acquired further resistance if the patient was being treated with the functional equivalent of only one drug for a significant period of time (usually considered to be 1 month or more). Depending on the drugs concerned, resistance sometimes develops if the patient was receiving the functional equivalent of two drugs. For example, pyrazinamide is not considered a good companion drug to prevent resistance (*1, 9*). If a patient was functionally receiving only rifampicin and pyrazinamide in the initial phase (because of resistance to isoniazid and ethambutol), resistance to rifampicin may develop.

7.11 Recording and reporting drug-resistant TB cases, evaluation of outcomes

Recording and reporting activities assist in the management of individual patients and enable managers to evaluate and improve the treatment outcomes of the programme as a whole. A system other than the standard one for drug-susceptible TB is recommended for drug-resistant TB cases. For registration of patients with drug resistance and for reporting treatment outcome for MDR patients, the reader is referred to reference *1*.

References

1. *Guidelines for the programmatic management of drug-resistant tuberculosis: emergency update 2008.* Geneva, World Health Organization, 2008 (WHO/HTM/TB/2008.402).
2. *International Standards for Tuberculosis Care (ISTC),* 2nd ed. The Hague, Tuberculosis Coalition for Technical Assistance, 2009.
3. *Molecular line probe assays for rapid screening of patients at risk of MDR-TB: policy statement.* Geneva, World Health Organization, 2008 (available at: www.who.int/tb/features_archive/policy_statement.pdf).
4. Sam IC et al. Mycobacterium tuberculosis and rifampin resistance, United Kingdom. *Emerging Infectious Diseases,* 2006, 12:752–759.

5. Suarez PG et al. Feasibility and cost-effectiveness of standardized second-line drug treatment for chronic tuberculosis patients: a national cohort study in Peru. *Lancet*, 2002, 359:1980–1989.

6. Resch SC et al. Cost-effectiveness of treating multidrug-resistant tuberculosis. *PLoS Medicine*, 2006, 3(7):e241.

7. Keshavjee S et al. Treatment of extensively drug-resistant tuberculosis in Tomsk, Russia: a retrospective cohort study. *Lancet*, 2008, 372:1403–1409.

8. Mitnick CD et al. Comprehensive treatment of extensively drug-resistant tuberculosis. *New England Journal of Medicine*, 2008, 359:563–574.

9. Mitchison DA. Basic mechanisms of chemotherapy. *Chest*, 1979, 76(6 Suppl.):771–781.

Treatment of extrapulmonary TB and of TB in special situations

8.1 Chapter objectives

This chapter describes:

— the treatment of extrapulmonary TB;
— important drug interactions;
— the treatment of TB in pregnancy and breastfeeding;
— the treatment of patients with pre-existing liver disease, renal failure or renal insufficiency.

8.2 Treatment of extrapulmonary TB

Although TB most commonly affects the lungs, any organ or tissue can be involved. In countries with comprehensive diagnostic and reporting systems, extrapulmonary TB accounts for 20–25% of reported cases. Globally, extrapulmonary cases (without concurrent pulmonary involvement) comprised 14% of notified cases (new and relapse) in 2007. Of specific forms of EPTB, lymphatic, pleural, and bone or joint disease are the most common, while pericardial, meningeal and disseminated (miliary) forms are more likely to result in a fatal outcome.

As discussed in Chapter 5, provider-initiated HIV testing is recommended as part of the evaluation of all TB patients and patients in whom the disease is suspected. HIV testing is especially important in persons with or suspected of having EPTB because of the increased frequency of extrapulmonary involvement in persons with immunosuppression. Extrapulmonary TB is considered to be WHO clinical stage 4 HIV disease (1). (More details on the treatment of TB in persons living with HIV are provided in Chapter 5.)

For WHO guidance on the prompt diagnosis of EPTB, see reference 1.

Pulmonary and extrapulmonary disease should be treated with the same regimens (see Chapter 3).[1] Note that some experts recommend 9–12 months of treatment for TB meningitis (2, 3) given the serious risk of disability and mortality, and 9 months of treatment for TB of bones or joints because of the difficulties of assessing treatment response (3). Unless drug resistance is suspected, adjuvant corticosteroid treatment is recommended for TB meningitis and pericarditis (1–4). In tuberculous meningitis, ethambutol should be replaced by streptomycin.

---

[1] This fourth edition no longer includes the option of omitting ethambutol during the intensive phase of treatment for patients with extrapulmonary disease who are known to be HIV-negative.

Although sometimes required for diagnosis, surgery plays little role in the treatment of extrapulmonary TB. It is reserved for management of late complications of disease such as hydrocephalus, obstructive uropathy, constrictive pericarditis and neurological involvement from Pott's disease (spinal TB). For large, fluctuant lymph nodes that appear to be about to drain spontaneously, aspiration or incision and drainage appear beneficial (3).

8.3 Important drug interactions

Many TB patients have concomitant illnesses. At the start of TB treatment, all patients should be asked about medicines they are currently taking. The most important interactions with anti-TB drugs are due to rifampicin. Rifampicin induces pathways that metabolize other drugs, thereby reducing the concentration and effect of those drugs. To maintain a therapeutic effect, dosages of the other drug(s) may need to be increased. When rifampicin is discontinued, its metabolism-inducing effect resolves within about 2 weeks, and dosages of the other drug(s) will need to be reduced (3).

More information on TB drug interactions is available in Annex 1 and on the web sites of the Global Drug Facility and the WHO Essential Medicines Library (www. stoptb.org/gdf/drugsupply/drugs_available.asp and www.who.int/emlib/Medicines. aspx).

Rifampicin substantially reduces the concentration and effect of the following drugs (for recommendations on dosage adjustment and on clinical or therapeutic drug monitoring, see reference 3):

— anti-infectives (including certain antiretroviral drugs discussed in section 5.6.1, mefloquine, azole antifungal agents, clarithromycin, erythromycin, doxycycline, atovaquone, chloramphenicol);
— hormone therapy,[1] including ethinylestradiol, norethindrone, tamoxifen, levothyroxine;
— methadone;
— warfarin;
— cyclosporin;
— corticosteroids;
— anticonvulsants (including phenytoin);
— cardiovascular agents including digoxin (among patients with renal insufficiency), digitoxin, verapamil, nifedipine, diltiazem, propranolol, metoprorol, enalapril, losartan, quinidine, mexiletine, tocainide, propafenone;
— theophylline;
— sulfonylurea hypoglycaemics;

---

[1] Rifampicin interacts with oral contraceptive medications leading to lowered protective efficacy. A woman receiving oral contraception may choose between two options while receiving treatment with rifampicin: following consultation with a clinician, an oral contraceptive pill containing a higher estrogen dose (50 µg), or another form of contraception.

— hypolipidaemics including simvastatin and fluvastatin;

— nortriptyline, haloperidol, quetiapine, benzodiazepines (including diazepam, triazolam), zolpidem, buspirone.

8.4 Treatment regimens in special situations

The treatment of TB in pregnancy and breastfeeding, liver disorders, and renal failure is discussed below.

8.4.1 Pregnancy and breastfeeding

Women of childbearing age should be asked about current or planned pregnancy before starting TB treatment. A pregnant woman should be advised that successful treatment of TB with the standard regimen is important for successful outcome of pregnancy. With the exception of streptomycin, the first line anti-TB drugs are safe for use in pregnancy: streptomycin is ototoxic to the fetus and should not be used during pregnancy.

A breastfeeding woman who has TB should receive a full course of TB treatment. Timely and properly applied chemotherapy is the best way to prevent transmission of tubercle bacilli to the baby. Mother and baby should stay together and the baby should continue to breastfeed. After active TB in the baby is ruled out, the baby should be given 6 months of isoniazid preventive therapy, followed by BCG vaccination (5).

Pyridoxine supplementation is recommended for all pregnant or breastfeeding women taking isoniazid (see section 4.8).

8.4.2 Liver disorders

This section covers TB treatment in patients with pre-existing liver disease; for detection and management of hepatitis induced by anti-TB drugs, see section 4.10.2.

Patients with the following conditions can receive the usual TB regimens provided that there is no clinical evidence of chronic liver disease: hepatitis virus carriage, a past history of acute hepatitis, current excessive alcohol consumption. However, hepatotoxic reactions to anti-TB drugs may be more common among these patients and should therefore be anticipated (see section 4.10.2).

In patients with unstable or advanced liver disease, liver function tests should be done at the start of treatment, if possible. If the serum alanine aminotransferase level (6) is more than 3 times normal before the initiation of treatment,[1] the following regimens should be considered (also discussed in section 4.10.2).[2] The more unstable or severe the liver disease is, the fewer hepatotoxic drugs should be used.

---

[1] Note that TB itself may involve the liver and cause abnormal liver function.

[2] In some cases of concurrent acute (i.e. viral) hepatitis not related to TB or TB treatment, it may be possible to defer TB treatment until the acute hepatitis has resolved.

Possible regimens include:

- Two hepatotoxic drugs (rather than the three in the standard regimen):
    — 9 months of isoniazid and rifampicin, plus ethambutol (until or unless isoniazid susceptibility is documented);
    — 2 months of isoniazid, rifampicin, streptomycin and ethambutol, followed by 6 months of isoniazid and rifampicin;
    — 6–9 months of rifampicin, pyrazinamide and ethambutol.

- One hepatotoxic drug:
    — 2 months of isoniazid, ethambutol and streptomycin, followed by 10 months of isoniazid and ethambutol.

- No hepatotoxic drugs:
    — 18–24 months of streptomycin, ethambutol and a fluoroquinolone.

Expert consultation is advisable in treating patients with advanced or unstable liver disease.

Clinical monitoring (and liver function tests, if possible) of all patients with pre-existing liver disease should be performed during treatment.

8.4.3   Renal failure and severe renal insufficiency

The recommended initial TB treatment regimen for patients with renal failure or severe renal insufficiency is 2 months of isoniazid, rifampicin, pyrazinamide and ethambutol, followed by 4 months of isoniazid and rifampicin. Isoniazid and rifampicin are eliminated by biliary excretion, so no change in dosing is necessary. There is significant renal excretion of ethambutol and metabolites of pyrazinamide, and doses should therefore be adjusted. Three times per week administration of these two drugs at the following doses is recommended: pyrazinamide (25 mg/kg), and ethambutol (15 mg/kg) (3, 7). These are the same mg/kg doses as those listed under Daily in Table 3.1.

While receiving isoniazid, patients with severe renal insufficiency or failure should also be given pyridoxine in order to prevent peripheral neuropathy (see section 4.8).

Because of an increased risk of nephrotoxicity and ototoxicity, streptomycin should be avoided in patients with renal failure. If streptomycin must be used, the dosage is 15 mg/kg, two or three times per week, to a maximum of 1 gram per dose, and serum levels of the drug should be monitored.

References

1. *Essential prevention and care interventions for adults and adolescents living with HIV in resource-limited settings.* Geneva, World Health Organization, 2008.

2. National Collaborating Centre for Chronic Conditions. *Tuberculosis: clinical diagnosis and management of tuberculosis, and measures for its prevention and control.* London, Royal College of Physicians, NICE (National Institute for Health and Clinical Excellence), 2006.

3. American Thoracic Society, CDC, Infectious Diseases Society of America. Treatment of tuberculosis. *Morbidity and Mortality Weekly Report: Recommendations and Reports*, 2003, 52(RR-11):1–77.

4. Thwaites GE et al. Dexamethasone for the treatment of tuberculous meningitis in adolescents and adults. *New England Journal of Medicine*, 2004, 351:1741–1751.

5. *Guidance for national tuberculosis programmes on the management of tuberculosis in children.* Geneva, World Health Organization, 2006 (WHO/HTM/TB/2006.371; WHO/FCH/CAH/2006.7).

6. Saukkonen JJ et al. An official ATS statement: hepatotoxicity of antituberculosis therapy. *American Journal of Respiratory and Critical Care Medicine*, 2006, 174:935–952.

7. *Guidelines for the programmatic management of drug-resistant tuberculosis: emergency update 2008.* Geneva, World Health Organization, 2008 (WHO/HTM/TB/2008.402).

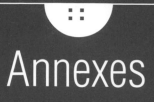

Annexes

A1

Essential first-line antituberculosis drugs[1]

Isoniazid

General information

Isoniazid, the hydrazide of isonicotinic acid, is highly bactericidal against replicating tubercle bacilli.

It is rapidly absorbed and diffuses readily into all fluids and tissues. The plasma half-life, which is genetically determined, varies from less than 1 hour in fast acetylators to more than 3 hours in slow acetylators. Isoniazid is largely excreted in the urine within 24 hours, mostly as inactive metabolites.

Clinical information

Administration and dosage
Isoniazid is normally taken orally but may be administered intramuscularly or intravenously to critically ill patients.

Adults:

5 mg/kg (4–6 mg/kg) daily, maximum 300 mg
10 mg/kg (8–12 mg/kg) three times weekly, maximum 900 mg (*1*).

Contraindications
- Known hypersensitivity.
- Active, unstable hepatic disease (with jaundice) – see section 8.4.2.

Precautions
Clinical monitoring (and liver function tests, if possible) should be performed during treatment of patients with pre-existing liver disease. Patients at risk of peripheral neuropathy, as a result of malnutrition, chronic alcohol dependence, HIV infection, pregnancy, breastfeeding, renal failure or diabetes, should additionally receive pyridoxine, 10 mg daily. Where the standard of health in the community is low, pyridoxine should be offered routinely. (Note that other guidelines (*1*) recommend a dose of 25 mg/day to prevent peripheral neuropathy). For established peripheral neuropathy, pyridoxine should be given at a larger dose of 50–75 mg daily (*2*).

---

[1] For drug preparations (include fixed-dose combinations) and costs, see the Global Drug Facility web site:
www.stoptb.org/gdf/drugsupply/drugs_available.asp. See also *WHO Model Formulary 2008*: www.who.int/selection_medicines/list/en/

Since isoniazid interacts with anticonvulsants used for epilepsy, it may be necessary to reduce the dosage of these drugs during treatment with isoniazid. If possible, serum concentrations of phenytoin and carbamazepine should be measured in patients receiving isoniazid with or without rifampicin (see *Drug interactions* below).

Use in pregnancy
Isoniazid is not known to be harmful in pregnancy (*3*). Pyridoxine supplementation is recommended for all pregnant (or breastfeeding) women taking isoniazid.

Adverse effects
Isoniazid is generally well tolerated at recommended doses.

Systemic or cutaneous hypersensitivity reactions occasionally occur during the first weeks of treatment.

Sleepiness or lethargy can be managed by reassurance or adjustment of the timing of administration.

The risk of peripheral neuropathy is excluded if vulnerable patients receive daily supplements of pyridoxine. Other less common forms of neurological disturbance, including optic neuritis, toxic psychosis and generalized convulsions, can develop in susceptible individuals, particularly in the later stages of treatment, and occasionally necessitate the withdrawal of isoniazid.

Symptomatic hepatitis is an uncommon but potentially serious reaction that can usually be averted by prompt withdrawal of treatment. More often, however, an asymptomatic rise in serum concentrations of hepatic transaminases at the outset of treatment is of no clinical significance and usually resolves spontaneously as treatment continues.

A lupus-like syndrome, pellagra, anaemia, and arthralgias are other rare adverse effects (*2*). Monoamine poisoning has been reported to occur after ingestion of foods and beverages with high monoamine content, but this is also rare (*1*).

Drug interactions
Isoniazid inhibits the metabolism of certain drugs, which can increase their plasma concentration to the point of toxicity. Rifampicin, however, has the opposite effect for many of these drugs. For example, the available data indicate that administering both rifampicin and isoniazid causes a reduction in plasma levels of phenytoin and diazepam (*1*).

Isoniazid may increase the toxicity of carbamazepine, benzodiazepines metabolized by oxidation (such as triazolam), acetaminophen, valproate, serotonergic antidepressants, disulfiram, warfarin and theophylline.

Overdosage

Nausea, vomiting, dizziness, blurred vision and slurring of speech occur within 30 minutes to 3 hours of overdosage. Massive poisoning results in coma preceded by respiratory depression and stupor. Severe intractable seizures may occur. Emesis and gastric lavage, activated charcoal, antiepileptics and IV sodium bicarbonate can be of value if instituted within a few hours of ingestion. Subsequently, haemodialysis may be of value. High doses of pyridoxine must be administered to prevent seizures.

Storage

Tablets should be kept in well-closed containers, protected from light. Solution for injection should be stored in ampoules, protected from light.

Rifampicin

General information

A semisynthetic derivative of rifamycin, rifampicin is a complex macrocyclic antibiotic that inhibits ribonucleic acid synthesis in a broad range of microbial pathogens. It has bactericidal action and a potent sterilizing effect against tubercle bacilli in both cellular and extracellular locations.

Rifampicin is lipid-soluble. Following oral administration, it is rapidly absorbed and distributed throughout the cellular tissues and body fluids; if the meninges are inflamed, significant amounts enter the cerebrospinal fluid. A single dose of 600 mg produces a peak serum concentration of about 10 µg/ml in 2–4 hours, which subsequently decays with a half-life of 2–3 hours. It is extensively recycled in the enterohepatic circulation, and metabolites formed by deacetylation in the liver are eventually excreted in the faeces.

Since resistance readily develops, rifampicin must always be administered in combination with other effective antimycobacterial agents.

Clinical information

Administration and dosage

Rifampicin should preferably be given at least 30 minutes before meals, since absorption is reduced when it is taken with food. However, this may not be clinically significant, and food can reduce intolerance to drugs. Rifampicin should always be given in combination with other effective antimycobacterial agents. It is also available for intravenous administration in critically ill patients (*1*).

Adults:

10 mg/kg (8–12 mg/kg) daily or 3 times weekly, maximum 600 mg.

Contraindications
- Known hypersensitivity to rifamycins.
- Active, unstable hepatic disease (with jaundice) – see section 8.4.2.

Precautions
Serious immunological reactions resulting in renal impairment, haemolysis or thrombocytopenia are on record in patients who resume taking rifampicin after a prolonged lapse of treatment. In this rare situation, rifampicin should be immediately and permanently withdrawn.

Clinical monitoring (and liver function tests, if possible) should be performed during treatment of all patients with pre-existing liver disease, who are at increased risk of further liver damage.

Patients should be warned that treatment may cause reddish coloration of all body secretions (urine, tears, saliva, sweat, semen and sputum), and that contact lenses and clothing may be irreversibly stained.

Use in pregnancy
Vitamin K should be administered at birth to the infant of a mother taking rifampicin because of the risk of postnatal haemorrhage.

Adverse effects
Rifampicin is well tolerated by most patients at currently recommended doses but may cause gastrointestinal reactions (abdominal pain, nausea, vomiting) and pruritus with or without rash (1).

Other adverse effects (fever, influenza-like syndrome and thrombocytopenia) are more likely to occur with intermittent administration.

Exfoliative dermatitis is more frequent in HIV-positive TB patients.

Temporary oliguria, dyspnoea and haemolytic anaemia have also been reported in patients taking the drug 3 times weekly; these reactions usually subside if the regimen is changed to daily dosage.

Moderate rises in serum concentrations of bilirubin and transaminases, which are common at the outset of treatment, are often transient and without clinical significance. However, dose-related hepatitis can occur and is potentially fatal: it is therefore important not to exceed the maximum recommended daily dose of 600 mg.

Drug interactions

Rifampicin induces hepatic enzymes, and may increase the dosage requirements of drugs metabolized in the liver (*1*), including:

— anti-infectives (including certain antiretroviral drugs discussed below and in section 5.6.1, mefloquine, azole antifungal agents, clarithromycin, erythromycin, doxycycline, atovaquone, chloramphenicol);
— hormone therapy, including ethinylestradiol, norethindrone, tamoxifen, levothyroxine;
— methadone;
— warfarin;
— cyclosporine;
— corticosteroids;
— anticonvulsants (including phenytoin);
— cardiovascular agents including digoxin (in patients with renal insufficiency), digitoxin, verapamil, nifedipine, diltiazem, propranolol, metoprorol, enalapril, losartan, quinidine, mexiletine, tocainide, propafenone;
— theophylline;
— sulfonylurea hypoglycaemics;
— hypolipidaemics including simvastatin and fluvastatin;
— nortriptyline, haloperidol, quetiapine, benzodiazepines (including diazepam, triazolam), zolpidem, buspirone.

Since rifampicin reduces the effectiveness of oral contraceptives, women should be advised to choose between one of two options for contraception. Following consultation with a clinician, the patient may use an oral contraceptive pill containing a higher dose of estrogen (50 µg); alternatively, a nonhormonal method of contraception may be used throughout rifampicin treatment and for at least one month subsequently.

Current antiretroviral drugs (non-nucleoside reverse transcriptase inhibitors and protease inhibitors) interact with rifampicin (see section 5.6.1). This may result in ineffectiveness of antiretroviral drugs, ineffective treatment of TB or an increased risk of drug toxicity.

Biliary excretion of radiocontrast media and sulfobromophthalein sodium may be reduced and microbiological assays for folic acid and vitamin B_{12} disturbed.

Overdosage

Gastric lavage may be of value if undertaken within a few hours of ingestion. Very large doses of rifampicin may depress central nervous function. There is no specific antidote and treatment is supportive.

Storage

Capsules and tablets should be kept in tightly closed containers, protected from light.

Pyrazinamide

General information

Pyrazinamide is a synthetic analogue of nicotinamide that is only weakly bactericidal against *M. tuberculosis* but has potent sterilizing activity, particularly in the relatively acidic intracellular environment of macrophages and in areas of acute inflammation. It is highly effective during the first 2 months of treatment while acute inflammatory changes persist. Its use has enabled treatment regimens to be shortened and the risk of relapse to be reduced.

It is readily absorbed from the gastrointestinal tract and is rapidly distributed throughout all tissues and fluids. Peak plasma concentrations are attained in 2 hours and the plasma half-life is about 10 hours. It is metabolized mainly in the liver and excreted largely in the urine.

Clinical information

Administration and dosage

Pyrazinamide is administered orally.

Adults (usually for the first 2 or 3 months of TB treatment):

25 mg/kg (20–30 mg/kg) daily
35 mg/kg (30–40 mg/kg) 3 times weekly.

Contraindications
- Known hypersensitivity.
- Active, unstable hepatic disease (with jaundice) – see Section 8.4.2.
- Porphyria.

Precautions

Patients with diabetes should be carefully monitored since blood glucose concentrations may become labile. Gout may be exacerbated. Clinical monitoring (and liver function tests, if possible) should be performed during treatment of patients with pre-existing liver disease. In patients with renal failure, pyrazinamide should be administered three times per week, rather than daily (see section 8.4.3 for doses).

Use in pregnancy

The 6-month regimen based upon isoniazid, rifampicin and pyrazinamide should be used whenever possible. Although detailed teratogenicity data are not available, pyrazinamide can probably be used safely during pregnancy (*1*).

Adverse effects

Pyrazinamide may cause gastrointestinal intolerance.

Hypersensitivity reactions are rare, but some patients complain of slight flushing of the skin.

Moderate rises in serum transaminase concentrations are common during the early phases of treatment. Severe hepatotoxicity is rare.

As a result of inhibition of renal tubular secretion, a degree of hyperuricaemia usually occurs, but this is often asymptomatic. Gout requiring treatment with allopurinol occasionally develops. Arthralgia, particularly of the shoulders, may occur and is responsive to simple analgesics (especially aspirin). Both hyperuricaemia and arthralgia may be reduced by prescribing regimens with intermittent administration of pyrazinamide.

Rare adverse events include sideroblastic anaemia (*2*) and photosensitive dermatitis (*1*).

Overdosage

Little has been recorded on the management of pyrazinamide overdose. Acute liver damage and hyperuricaemia have been reported. Treatment is essentially symptomatic. Emesis and gastric lavage may be of value if undertaken within a few hours of ingestion. There is no specific antidote and treatment is supportive.

Storage

Tablets should be stored in tightly closed containers, protected from light.

Streptomycin

General information

Streptomycin is an aminoglycoside antibiotic derived from *Streptomyces griseus* that is used in the treatment of TB and sensitive Gram-negative infections.

Streptomycin is not absorbed from the gastrointestinal tract but, after intramuscular administration, it diffuses readily into the extracellular component of most body tissues and attains bactericidal concentrations, particularly in tuberculous cavities. Little normally enters the cerebrospinal fluid, although penetration increases when the meninges are inflamed. The plasma half-life, which is normally 2–3 hours, is considerably extended in the newborn, the elderly and patients with severe renal impairment. Streptomycin is excreted unchanged in the urine.

Clinical information

Administration and dosage

Streptomycin must be administered by deep intramuscular injection. Syringes and needles should be adequately sterilized to exclude any risk of transmitting viral pathogens. It is also available for intravenous administration (*1*).

Adults:

> 15 mg/kg (12–18 mg/kg) daily, or 2 or 3 times weekly;
> maximum daily dose is 1000 mg.

Patients aged over 60 years may not be able to tolerate more than 500–750 mg daily, so some guidelines recommend reducing the dose to 10 mg/kg per day for patients in this age group (*1*). Patients weighing less than 50 kg may not tolerate doses above 500–750 mg daily.[1]

Contraindications

- Known hypersensitivity.
- Auditory nerve impairment.
- Myasthenia gravis.
- Pregnancy.

Precautions

Hypersensitivity reactions are rare. If they do occur (usually during the first weeks of treatment), streptomycin should be withdrawn immediately. Once fever and skin rash have resolved, desensitization may be attempted.

Both the elderly and patients with renal impairment are vulnerable to dose-related toxic effects resulting from accumulation. Streptomycin should be used with caution in patients with renal insufficiency, because of the increased risk of nephrotoxicity and ototoxicity. The dose should be maintained at 12–15 mg/kg but at a reduced frequency of 2–3 times per week (*1*). Where possible, serum levels should be monitored periodically and dosage adjusted appropriately to ensure that plasma concentrations, as measured when the next dose is due, do not exceed 4 µg/ml.

Protective gloves should be worn when streptomycin injections are administered, to avoid sensitization dermatitis.

Use in pregnancy

Streptomycin should not be used in pregnancy: it crosses the placenta and can cause auditory nerve impairment and nephrotoxicity in the fetus.

---

[1] *WHO Essential Medicines Library* (http://apps.who.int/emlib/MedicineDisplay.aspx?Language=EN&MedIDName=310%40streptomycin; accessed January 2010).

Adverse effects
Streptomycin injections are painful. Rash, induration, or sterile abscesses can form at injection sites.

Numbness and tingling around the mouth occur immediately after injection.

Cutaneous hypersensitivity reactions can occur.

Impairment of vestibular function is uncommon with currently recommended doses. Hearing loss is less common than vertigo. Manifestations of damage to the 8th cranial (auditory) nerve include ringing in the ears, ataxia, vertigo and deafness; damage usually occurs in the first 2 months of treatment and is reversible if the dosage is reduced or the drug is stopped (2).

Streptomycin is less nephrotoxic than other aminoglycoside antibiotics. If urinary output falls, albuminuria occurs or tubular casts are detected in the urine, streptomycin should be stopped and renal function should be evaluated.

Haemolytic anaemia, aplastic anaemia, agranulocytosis, thrombocytopenia and lupoid reactions are rare adverse effects.

Drug interactions
Other ototoxic or nephrotoxic drugs should not be administered to patients receiving streptomycin. These include other aminoglycoside antibiotics, amphotericin B, cefalosporins, etacrynic acid, cyclosporin, cisplatin, furosemide and vancomycin.

Streptomycin may potentiate the effect of neuromuscular blocking agents administered during anaesthesia.

Overdosage
Haemodialysis can be beneficial. There is no specific antidote and treatment is supportive.

Storage
Solutions retain their potency for 48 hours after reconstitution at room temperature and for up to 14 days when refrigerated. Powder for injection should be stored in tightly closed containers, protected from light.

Ethambutol

General information

A synthetic congener of 1,2-ethanediamine, ethambutol is active against *M. tuberculosis*, *M. bovis* and some nonspecific mycobacteria. It is used in combination with other anti-TB drugs to prevent or delay the emergence of resistant strains.

It is readily absorbed from the gastrointestinal tract. Plasma concentrations peak in 2–4 hours and decay with a half-life of 3–4 hours. Ethambutol is excreted in the urine both unchanged and as inactive hepatic metabolites. About 20% is excreted unchanged in the faeces.

Clinical information

Administration and dosage

Ethambutol is administered orally.

Adults:

15 mg/kg (15–20 mg/kg) daily

30 mg/kg (25–35 mg/kg) 3 times weekly.

Dosage must always be carefully calculated on a weight basis to avoid toxicity, and the dose or the dosing interval should be adjusted in patients with impaired renal function (creatinine clearance <70 ml/min). If creatinine clearance is less than 30 ml/minute, ethambutol should be administered 3 times per week (see section 8.4.3) (1).

Contraindications

- Known hypersensitivity.
- Pre-existing optic neuritis from any cause.

Precautions

Patients should be advised to discontinue treatment immediately and to report to a clinician if their sight or perception of colour deteriorates. Ocular examination is recommended before and during treatment (3). Whenever possible, renal function should be assessed before treatment. Plasma ethambutol concentration should be monitored if creatinine clearance is less than 30 ml/min.

Use in pregnancy

Ethambutol is not known to be harmful in pregnancy (3).

Adverse effects

Dose-dependent optic neuritis can result in impairment of visual acuity and colour vision in one or both eyes. Early changes are usually reversible, but blindness can occur if treatment is not discontinued promptly. Ocular toxicity is rare when ethambutol is used for 2–3 months at recommended doses.

Signs of peripheral neuritis occasionally develop in the legs.

Other rare adverse events include generalized cutaneous reaction, arthralgia and, very rarely, hepatitis.

Overdosage

Emesis and gastric lavage may be of value if undertaken within a few hours of ingestion. Subsequently, dialysis may be of value. There is no specific antidote and treatment is supportive.

Storage

Tablets should be stored in tightly closed containers.

References

1. American Thoracic Society, CDC, Infectious Diseases Society of America. Treatment of tuberculosis. *Morbidity and Mortality Weekly Report: Recommendations and Reports*, 2003,52(RR-11):1–77.
2. Toman K. *Toman's tuberculosis. Case detection, treatment, and monitoring: questions and answers*, 2nd ed. Geneva, World Health Organization, 2004.
3. *WHO Model Formulary 2008*. Geneva, World Health Organization, 2009 (available at www.who.int/selection_medicines/list/WMF2008.pdf).

Summary of evidence and considerations underlying the recommendations

With input from the Guidelines Group, WHO finalized a list of seven key questions on the treatment of TB. Systematic literature reviews were conducted for each question and the evidence was synthesized.

The evidence is summarized for each question and is followed by a description of the benefits, harms, and other considerations used in developing the recommendations and rating them as strong or conditional using the GRADE system (See Chapter 1, section 1.6 for a description of the methodology, including definitions of "strong", "conditional" and "weak"). At the time of publication of this fourth edition, evidence gathered through some of the systematic reviews had not been published.[1]

Some of the remarks listed in the Executive Summary under each recommendation are included in the Other considerations section for each question below. Where evidence is lacking, future research is suggested (Annex 5).

Question 1. Duration of rifampicin

Should new pulmonary TB patients be treated with the 6-month or the 2-month rifampicin regimen?

Summary of evidence

A systematic review and meta-analysis included 21 472 participants in 312 arms of 57 randomized controlled trials (RCTs) conducted in various regions of the world since 1965 (1). In three of the 57 trials, patients were randomly assigned to either a 2-month rifampicin or a 6-month rifampicin arm; rates of failure, relapse and acquired drug resistance were compared "head-to-head" across the two study arms. In a multivariate regression analysis, each arm of the 57 RCTs was treated as a separate cohort, and results were adjusted for potentially confounding patient and treatment factors.

Benefits and harms of changing to the 6-month rifampicin regimen

The three studies with head-to-head comparisons showed that the risk of relapse after a 6-month rifampicin regimen was significantly lower than that after a 2-month rifampicin regimen. If a country were to change from a 2-month to a 6-month rifampicin regimen, the benefit would be an estimated 112 relapses averted per 1000 TB patients.

---

[1] GRADE tables for unpublished evidence are available from WHO upon request.

Regression analysis suggests that changing to a 6-month regimen would significantly reduce failure and acquired drug resistance rates, in addition to relapse rates.[1] This analysis found that regimens with 5–7 months of rifampicin have 0.43 times the failure rate of those with 1–2 months of rifampicin, and 0.32 times the relapse rate. Among the failures and relapses from regimens with 5–7 months of rifampicin, the rate of acquired drug resistance is 0.28 times that of the regimens with 1–2 months of rifampicin.

Patients with isoniazid resistance would realize major benefits if the 2-month rifampicin regimen were replaced with a 6-month regimen. Among patients with isoniazid mono-resistance at the start of treatment, 38% relapsed after treatment with 2-month rifampicin regimens, which is significantly higher than the 5.5% relapse rate after treatment with 6-month rifampicin regimens. Thus, changing to the 6-month rifampicin regimen would avert 325 relapses per 1000 patients[2] who start treatment with isoniazid resistance.

Even for patients with pan-susceptible TB, the proportion who relapsed after the 2-month rifampicin regimen was 8.2%, significantly higher than the 3.1% for the 6-month rifampicin regimen.

When the first course of therapy is considered along with retreatment for patients who fail or relapse, it is estimated that the 6-month rifampicin regimen would avert between 3 and 12 deaths per 1000 compared with the 2-month rifampicin regimen across 7 countries modelled with a range of drug resistance among new patients. In addition, 0.6–4.4 failures and relapses with drug resistance other than MDR would be averted per 1000 TB patients, but an additional 0.6–1.3 MDR-TB cases would be generated.

Among patients who failed or relapsed after their first course of treatment containing 6 months of rifampicin, regression analysis found a reduction in overall acquired drug resistance; however, the pattern of acquired drug resistance was different from that in patients who received the 2-month rifampicin regimen. The risk of acquiring drug resistance other than MDR is higher with the 2-month rifampicin regimen, but the risk of acquiring MDR is higher with the 6-month rifampicin regimen. Among failures, the proportion with MDR is predicted to be 4–56% after initial treatment with the 2-month rifampicin regimen but 50–94% after initial treatment with the regimen containing 6 months of rifampicin.

Other considerations

To help minimize the acquisition of MDR, it is critically important that NTPs ensure adequate supervision of rifampicin. Implementing patient supervision for the 4-month continuation phase will require additional resources in areas where the

---

[1] The difference in failure and acquired drug resistance was not statistically significant in these three RCTs.

[2] 38 minus 5.5 per 100 = 325 per 1000.

continuation phase has been self-administered – an investment that may be offset by the savings from relapses (and therefore retreatments) averted. In 2008, 23 countries (including 4 that are considered high-burden) still used the 2-month rifampicin regimen for their new patients. These countries reported 706 905 new cases in 2007, or 13% of the global new TB notifications that year. Another resource consideration is the fact that when purchased through the Global Drug Facility, a 2HRZE/4HR patient kit is US$ 4–10 less expensive than a 2HRZE/6HE kit.

The interactions of rifampicin with antiretroviral therapy (ART) are of concern. Switching to the 6-month rifampicin regimen means that these drug interactions must be taken into account for the full 6 months rather than for just the first 2 months of therapy. However, the 6-month rifampicin regimen has marked benefits for persons living with HIV (see Question 4 below), and the drug interactions can be managed (see section 5.6.1). Moreover, ART is often initiated during the first 2 months of TB therapy when treatment regimens include rifampicin.

It was assumed that all patients prefer a regimen that saves lives.

Conclusion

Recommendations 1.1 and 1.2 place high value on saving lives. Given both the high quality of evidence for this benefit and the fact that the potential harm of acquired MDR can be mitigated by supervision of treatment (and possibly with a modified regimen for new patients in areas with high levels of isoniazid resistance), these are both strong recommendations. Periodic drug resistance surveys (or ongoing surveillance) in each country are essential for monitoring the impact of the regimen and the overall treatment programme.

■ **Recommendation 1.1**
   New patients with pulmonary TB should receive a regimen containing 6 months of rifampicin: 2HRZE/4HR

   (Strong/High grade of evidence)

■ **Recommendation 1.2**
   The 2HRZE/6HE treatment regimen should be phased out

   (Strong/High grade of evidence)

Question 2. Frequency of dosing in new patients

When a country selects 2HRZE/4HR, should patients be treated daily or three times weekly during the intensive phase?

Summary of evidence

A systematic review and meta-analysis included 21 472 participants in 312 arms of 57 randomized controlled trials (RCTs) conducted in various regions of the world since

1965 (*1*). In a multivariate regression analysis, each arm of the 57 RCTs was treated as a separate cohort, and results were adjusted for potentially confounding patient and treatment factors. Only one study of 223 patients evaluated a rifampicin-containing regimen administered twice weekly throughout therapy; this study was not included in the meta-analyses.

Benefits and harms of intermittent dosing

No significant increase in failure, relapse or acquired drug resistance was found when daily dosing throughout therapy was compared with the following intermittent regimens in new TB patients overall:

— daily then three times weekly;
— daily then twice weekly; or
— three times weekly throughout therapy.

However, the regression analysis showed that patients being treated three times weekly throughout therapy rates of acquired drug resistance that were 3.3 times higher than those in patients who received daily drug administration throughout treatment.

The meta-analysis revealed no difference in rates of failure, relapse or acquired drug resistance in pan-susceptible new patients being treated with these dosing schedules. However, use of a three times weekly intensive phase schedule in patients with pretreatment isoniazid resistance was associated with a significantly higher risk of failure and acquired drug resistance in another meta-analysis (see Question 3).

Other considerations

When based in a health facility, daily administration of therapy places a larger burden on TB programmes and patients than intermittent therapy. Intermittent regimens require stronger programmes with higher quality patient supervision, but all regimens should be provided with full patient supervision and support (see Chapter 6).

Studies of patients' preferences for dosing schedules were not systematically reviewed.

The higher isoniazid dose used in intermittent therapy was not considered to have an increased incidence of adverse effects. (The rifampicin dosage is unchanged when using intermittent therapy.)

In an international, multicentre, randomized trial (Union Study A), Jindani, Nunn & Enarson found three times weekly dosing resulted in significantly lower culture conversion rates at 2 months (*2*). In developing recommendations, this end-point was ranked as important but not critical for decision-making (Annex 3), and was not part of the systematic review.

Conclusion

For new patients without HIV infection, high-quality evidence demonstrated no significant difference in regimens that were administered daily throughout, daily initially then intermittently in the continuation phase, or three times weekly throughout treatment.

Daily[1] dosing is optimal because it probably achieves better adherence under programme conditions. In addition, meta-analyses showed the superiority of daily (compared with three times weekly) intensive-phase dosing for patients with pretreatment isoniazid resistance and for preventing acquired drug resistance in patients overall.

Given the above considerations of these schedules, Recommendation 2 for daily dosing throughout therapy is strong; three times weekly intermittent regimens, which were found to be equally efficacious,[2] are listed as alternatives to daily treatment throughout therapy.

There are insufficient data to support the use of regimens that are given twice weekly throughout therapy. On operational grounds, twice weekly dosing is not recommended since missing one dose means the patient receives only half the regimen. The recommendation against the use of this regimen is therefore rated as strong.

■ **Recommendation 2.1**

   Wherever feasible, the optimal dosing frequency for new patients with pulmonary TB is daily throughout the course of therapy

   (Strong/High grade of evidence)

There are two alternatives to Recommendation 2.1:

   ■ **Recommendation 2.1A**

   New patients with pulmonary TB may receive a daily intensive phase followed by three times weekly continuation phase [2HRZE/4(HR)$_3$], provided that each dose is directly observed

   (Conditional/High or moderate grade of evidence))

   ■ **Recommendation 2.1B**

   Three times weekly dosing throughout therapy [2(HRZE)$_3$/4(HR)$_3$], provided that every dose is directly observed therapy and the patient is NOT living with HIV or living in an HIV-prevalent setting

   (Conditional/High or moderate grade of evidence)

---

[1] While the definition of the term varies across countries, "daily" is considered to mean at least five times per week.
[2] Three times per week regimens are delivered in a variety of schedules across countries.

■ **Recommendation 2.2**

New patients with TB should not receive twice weekly dosing for the full course of treatment unless this is done in the context of formal research

(Strong/High grade of evidence)

Question 3. Initial regimen in countries with high levels of isoniazid resistance

In countries with high levels of isoniazid resistance in new TB patients, should the continuation phase (containing isoniazid and rifampicin) be changed in the standard treatment of all new patients, in order to prevent the development of multidrug resistance? (This question applies to countries where isoniazid susceptibility testing in new patients is not done – or results are not available – before the continuation phase begins.)

Summary of evidence

The systematic review described in Questions 1 and 2 revealed that, when receiving a regimen including 5-7 months of rifampicin, patients with pretreatment isoniazid resistance (but susceptibility to rifampicin and streptomycin) were 22 times more likely to acquire drug resistance than patients who started treatment with drug-susceptible disease (1).

A systematic review and meta-analysis was conducted of 33 trials involving 1907 new and previously treated patients with isoniazid monoresistance.[1] The use of at least three effective drugs during the continuation phase was associated with a significantly lower risk of failure, and the use of four or more effective drugs during the intensive phase was associated with a significantly lower risk of failure, relapse and acquired drug resistance. The use of a daily intensive phase was associated with a significantly lower risk of failure and acquired drug resistance. The use of streptomycin was associated with a significantly lower risk of failure and acquired drug resistance. The risk of relapse was significantly lower with the use of 6 months of rifampicin compared with 2 months, and 5 months of pyrazinamide compared with no pyrazinamide.

Benefits and harms of adding ethambutol to the continuation phase

The addition of ethambutol was considered as an intervention to avoid what would, in effect, be monotherapy in the continuation phase of new patients with isoniazid resistance (3). Surveillance data show that only 0.6% of new patients have resistance to both ethambutol and isoniazid, indicating that the regimen has potential efficacy (4).

---

[1] Manuscript was submitted, but not published at the time of publication of this document. GRADE tables are available from WHO upon request.

A few potential harms are associated with the addition of ethambutol to the continuation phase of rifampicin and isoniazid. In countries where the level of isoniazid resistance in new patients equals the global weighted mean of 7.4%, 74 TB patients per 1000 will have isoniazid resistance. This means that for every 1000 new TB patients, 926 patients with isoniazid-susceptible TB will receive ethambutol unnecessarily in order to treat the 74 with isoniazid resistance. The risk of ocular toxicity due to ethambutol was not systematically reviewed for this edition.

While widespread use of ethambutol could increase the risk of acquired ethambutol resistance, ethambutol is not as critical as the injectables or fluoroquinolones for the treatment of MDR-TB. The acquisition of ethambutol resistance is less harmful than the acquisition of resistance to the two classes of drugs that form the backbone of MDR-TB regimens. However, loss of a less toxic drug (if the MDR strain retains susceptibility) may jeopardize the ability to cure MDR-TB.

Other considerations

The existence of a fixed-dose combination of isoniazid, ethambutol and rifampicin makes the addition of ethambutol operationally feasible. Countries can use their drug resistance survey data in new patients to determine whether the level of isoniazid resistance in new patients warrants the addition of ethambutol.[1] However, about 50% of countries (including four high-burden countries) have no drug resistance surveillance data, even at a subnational level (*1*).[2]

Several alternatives to ethambutol were considered, but rejected, as means to "protect rifampicin" in patients with pre-treatment isoniazid resistance:

- The meta-analysis showed that treatment for 5 or more months with pyrazinamide is associated with a significant decrease in relapse but is not associated with a lower risk of acquired drug resistance. Although data on adverse effects were not systematically reviewed, pyrazinamide can cause hepatotoxicity (particularly when administered with antiretroviral therapy). Pyrazinamide-associated joint pain can lead to poor adherence.

- While likely to be effective in preventing acquired drug resistance, the use of a fluoroquinolone in the continuation phase for all new patients would jeopardize this critical class of drugs for MDR-TB patients.

- A sputum smear obtained after the second month of treatment is not helpful for detecting pretreatment isoniazid resistance (Question 5).

---

[1] Annex 1 (p. 121) of the 4th WHO/IUATLD Anti-TB Drug Resistance Project displays each country s most recent drug resistance survey results in new patients. To determine the level of any isoniazid resistance (excluding MDR), countries will need to do the following calculation: % any isoniazid resistance (column 12) minus % MDR (column 30). This annex is available at: www.who.int/tb/features_ archive/drsreport_launch_26feb08/en/index.html.

[2] Sample sizes in WHO-sponsored drug resistance surveys are sufficiently large to allow precise countrywide estimates, but not estimates for subregions or populations (unless they were specifically sampled).

Conclusion

This recommendation places a high value on preventing the development of MDR in areas where isoniazid resistance is prevalent among new cases and isoniazid susceptibility testing in new patients is not done (or results are not available) before the continuation phase begins. It is a conditional recommendation for the following reasons.

The most effective regimen for the treatment of isoniazid-resistant TB is not known. There is inadequate evidence to quantify the ability of ethambutol to "protect rifampicin" in patients with pre-treatment isoniazid resistance. There is a risk of permanent blindness, although evidence for ocular toxicity from ethambutol was not systematically reviewed for this edition.

Further research (see Annex 5) is thus needed to define the level of isoniazid resistance that would warrant the addition of ethambutol (or other drugs) to the continuation phase of the standard regimen for new patients in TB programmes where isoniazid susceptibility testing in new patients is not done (or results are not available) before the continuation phase begins.

See also Question 2: In patients with pretreatment isoniazid resistance, daily dosing during the intensive phase was associated with significantly lower risks of failure and acquired drug resistance than three times weekly dosing during the intensive phase.

■ **Recommendation 3**

   In populations with known or suspected high levels of isoniazid resistance, new TB patients may receive HRE as therapy in the continuation phase as an acceptable alternative to HR

   (Weak/Insufficient evidence, expert opinion)

Question 4. TB treatment in persons living with HIV

Should intermittent regimens be used for persons living with HIV? What should be the duration of TB treatment in people living with HIV?

Summary of evidence

A systematic review and meta-analysis of 6 randomized controlled trials and 23 cohort studies provided pooled estimates of failure, relapse and death by duration of rifampicin, and daily intensive phase vs intermittent throughout (5). The systematic review revealed a marked and significant reduction in failure and relapse in the arms where some or all patients received ART.

Benefits and harms of intermittent intensive phase, and of extending the duration of therapy

In a regression model, treatment failure or relapse was 1.8–2.5 times more likely with intermittent rather than daily dosing in the intensive phase.

Compared with 8 or more months of rifampicin, 2-month rifampicin regimens carried a 3-fold higher risk of relapse and 6-month regimens a 2.2 -fold higher risk.

Other considerations and conclusions

Because most of the data in the systematic review are from cohort studies, the data quality is considered low. Nonetheless, daily dosing during the intensive phase is a strong recommendation for people living with HIV for the following reasons:

- The investment in changing from intermittent to daily therapy during the intensive phase represents a wise use of resources given the potential benefit.

- Patients are assumed to prefer a regimen with lower failure and relapse, even if they have to come to a health facility for daily dosing.

The meta-analysis of TB patients living with HIV contained no data comparing a daily with a three times weekly continuation phase. For this reason, and for consistency with Recommendation 2.1, Recommendations 4.2 and 4.3 are conditional.

Extending treatment beyond 6 months is recommended by some expert groups in certain persons living with HIV (6) and the meta-analysis showed that this is associated with significantly lower relapse rates (5). However, several other considerations are given greater weight. Separate regimens for TB patients living with or without HIV would be operationally very challenging and could add stigma. Other potential harms of extending treatment are acquired rifampicin resistance, and a longer period during which antiretroviral therapy options are limited (because of ART–rifampicin interactions).

■ **Recommendation 4.1**

TB patients with known positive HIV status and all TB patients living in HIV-prevalent settings[1] should receive daily TB treatment at least during the intensive phase

(Strong/High grade of evidence)

■ **Recommendation 4.2**

For the continuation phase, the optimal dosing frequency is also daily for these patients

(Strong/High grade of evidence)

---

[1] HIV-prevalent settings are defined as countries, subnational administrative units, or selected facilities where the HIV prevalence among adult pregnant women is ≥1% or HIV prevalence among TB patients is ≥5% (7).

■ **Recommendation 4.3**

If a daily continuation phase is not possible for these patients, three times weekly dosing during the continuation phase is an acceptable alternative

(Conditional/High or moderate grade of evidence)

■ **Recommendation 4.4**

It is recommended that TB patients who are living with HIV receive the same duration of TB treatment as HIV-negative TB patients

(Strong/High grade of evidence)

Question 5. Sputum monitoring during TB treatment of smear-positive pulmonary TB patients

In pulmonary TB patients who are initially smear-positive, how effective are sputum specimens for predicting relapse, failure and pretreatment isoniazid resistance?

Summary of findings

To determine the ability of sputum smears at months 2 or 3 of treatment to predict relapse, results of randomized controlled trials conducted by the British Medical Research Council (MRC) involving approximately 1900 patients from the 1970s and 80s across Asia and east Africa were reanalysed.[1] All patients received a 6-month regimen with at least four drugs in the initial 2 months. The sensitivity of the smear at either month 2 or month 3 in identifying patients who will relapse is less than 40%; less than one-quarter of the patients with positive smears will relapse (assuming a 7% relapse rate).

A separate systematic review[2] also found that sputum smear at month 2 or 3 of treatment has limited utility in predicting relapse. For evaluating a diagnostic test (7), the MRC reanalysis and the systematic review are considered moderate- and low-quality evidence, respectively.

It is not possible to determine the ability of the smear to predict failure for the following reasons:

• In the MRC trials, there were few treatment failures observed and it was therefore impossible to carry out a meaningful analysis.

• In the systematic review, the quality of evidence in most studies that assessed failure is very low.

---

[1] The original published results from these studies were based on analyses using per-protocol populations. The reanalysis was based on individual patient, intention-to-treat data. All cultures were done on solid media.

[2] Manuscript was not published at the time of publication of this document. GRADE tables are available from WHO upon request.

Benefits and harms of obtaining a smear at 3 months and, if positive, obtaining culture and DST

The main rationale for recommending the addition of a 3-month sputum smear is to detect poor response to therapy earlier than the fifth month (the current algorithm). High value was placed on the need to detect MDR as soon as possible, even though the MRC reanalysis showed that smear or culture results at month 1, 2, 3 or 4 are not predictive of pretreatment isoniazid resistance. (The MRC studies were done before the emergence of rifampicin resistance and are therefore not directly relevant to the ability of sputum monitoring to detect MDR-TB.)

The alternative of using the 2-month smear for triggering a culture was also considered. The advantage would be earlier detection of MDR-TB (since most will have had no DST at the start of therapy). However, there are programmatic benefits from using the 3-month (rather than the 2-month) smear as a trigger for culture and DST. For every 1000 TB patients who are smear-positive at the start of treatment, 183 are expected to remain smear-positive at 2 months and only 83 at 3 months. By intervening with culture and DST on the basis of the 3-month, rather than the 2-month, sputum smear result, national TB programmes will have 100 fewer patients needing these more complex laboratory tests for every 1000 TB patients who start therapy.

Other considerations and conclusion

These recommendations retain the original purpose of sputum monitoring, which was to assess programme performance. High value is placed on the need to detect treatment failure due to MDR-TB earlier in the course of treatment than the fifth month (as per the previous WHO algorithm). Given the moderate to low quality of evidence and operational concerns arising from the poor ability of the smear to predict relapse, this is a conditional recommendation.

■ **Recommendation 5.1**

For smear-positive pulmonary TB patients treated with first-line drugs, sputum smear microscopy may be performed at completion of the intensive phase of treatment

(Conditional/High or moderate grade of evidence)

■ **Recommendation 5.2**

In new patients, if the specimen obtained at the end of the intensive phase (month 2) is smear-positive, sputum smear microscopy should optimally be obtained at the end of the month 3

(Strong/High grade of evidence)

■ **Recommendation 5.3**

In new patients, if the specimen obtained at the end of month 3 is smear-positive, sputum culture and drug susceptibility testing (DST) should be performed

(Strong/High grade of evidence)

■ **Recommendation 5.4**

In previously treated patients, if the specimen obtained at the end of the intensive phase (month 3) is smear-positive, sputum culture and drug susceptibility testing (DST) should be performed

(Strong/High grade of evidence)

Question 6. Treatment extension in new pulmonary TB patients

In new pulmonary TB patients, how effective is extension of treatment for preventing failure or relapse?

Summary of findings

The systematic review identified only one relevant study.[1] A study currently under way in Bangladesh of a 6-month rifampicin-containing regimen randomized 3775 new smear-positive patients who remained positive at 2 months to either the 1-month extension arm (extension of the intensive phase by 1 month) or the no-extension arm.

Benefits and risks of extending treatment for patients who are smear-positive at 2 months

Preliminary results at 1 year of follow-up showed that patients in the 1-month extension arm had a significantly lower relapse rate (relative risk 0.37, 95% CI 0.21, 0.66) than patients in the no-extension arm. A smaller decrease in failure in the 1-month extension arm was not statistically significant. Given the preliminary nature of the results and passive follow up of patients, the evidence from the Bangladesh study was graded moderate quality.

In 1000 TB patients with a 7% risk of relapse, the Bangladesh study predicts that extending the treatment of 183 patients who are smear-positive at 2 months would avert 16 of the 70 expected relapses.[2] However, to achieve this 23% reduction in relapses, 158 patients per 1000 would be incorrectly predicted to relapse; their treatment would be extended unnecessarily.

---

[1] GRADE tables are available from WHO upon request.

[2] Estimates from Question 5 shows that the 2-month smear will correctly identify 25 patients who will relapse after treatment and incorrectly identify 158 patients who will not relapse) If the intensive phase is extended for these 25 patients whose positive smear at 2 months correctly predicts that they will relapse, the Bangladesh study predicts that they will have a 37% reduction in relapse. Instead of all 25 relapsing, only 9 per 1000 would relapse (0.37 x 25); that is, 16 relapses would be prevented. Hence, instead of the 70 expected relapses in the cohort of 1000, obtaining sputum smears at 2 months and extending treatment for those who are smear-positive would result in 54 relapses, a 23% reduction.

Other considerations and conclusion

While extending rifampicin beyond 6 months reduces the risk of relapse,[1] there is insufficient evidence to determine which patients are most likely to benefit. Historically, when the new patient regimen included only 2 months of rifampicin, the extension of the intensive phase meant an extra month of supervised rifampicin. This extra month is less important now, when the recommended regimen is 6 months of supervised rifampicin. Given these considerations, together with preliminary results from one moderate-quality study that showed only modest benefit, a conditional recommendation was made not to extend treatment on the basis of a positive smear at 2 months.

■ **Recommendation 6**

   In patients treated with the regimen containing rifampicin throughout treatment, if a positive sputum smear is found at completion of the intensive phase, extension of the intensive phase is not recommended

   (Strong/High grade of evidence)

Question 7. Previously treated patients

Which (if any) groups of patients should receive a retreatment regimen with first-line drugs?

Summary of findings

The systematic review found no randomized controlled trial of the 8-month retreatment regimen with first-line drugs. Six cohort studies of this regimen in previously treated patients included 898 with pan-susceptible strains and 124 with isoniazid monoresistance. Failure rates ranged from 1% to 27% in patients with pan-susceptible disease and from 18% to 44% in those with isoniazid monorcsistance (8).

In developing recommendations, the retreatment regimen of first-line drugs was considered only for empirical therapy, while awaiting DST results, previously treated patients at medium to low likelihood of MDR.[2] However, the recommendations are not rated since the quality of evidence was not evaluated according to GRADE methodology.

---

[1] The head-to-head comparison described in Question 1 showed a 4% difference between the proportion relapsing after 6 months of rifampicin-containing treatment and the proportion relapsing after 9 months of rifampicin-containing treatment.

[2] Countries that adopt rapid DST (such as the line probe assay) will be able to confirm or exclude MDR within hours to days. This allows the results to guide the choice of regimen right at the start of treatment. These countries do not need the retreatment regimen with first-line drugs. Countries using conventional DST will need an empirical MDR regimen for previously treated patients with a high likelihood of having MDR, while awaiting DST results. For those with a medium or low likelihood of having MDR-TB, the benefits and harms of using of the 8-month retreatment regimen with first-line drugs (while awaiting DST results) are as discussed in the text.

Benefits and harms of using a retreatment regimen with first-line drugs for patients with low to medium likelihood of having MDR

For retreatment of patients who do not have MDR, the first-line drug retreatment regimen avoids exposure to a prolonged regimen of toxic second-line drugs. Other benefits for non-MDR patients are savings in patient time and resources and, probably, a diminished risk of defaulting. By using only first-line drugs, the WHO retreatment regimen conserves programme resources and preserves the activity of fluoroquinolones and injectables (amikacin and kanamycin) for patients who truly need these drugs (i.e. those with documented MDR).

On a global level, 65% of previously treated patients have *M. tuberculosis* organisms that are still fully susceptible (4). For these patients, the first-line retreatment regimen provides the benefit of the two best anti-TB drugs, isoniazid and rifampicin. For the 12.4% of previously treated patients at the global level whose *M. tuberculosis* is isoniazid-resistant but not MDR, the retreatment regimen of first-line drugs is of unproven efficacy; however, the data in Question 3 suggest that the use of streptomycin, a daily intensive phase, and four effective drugs in the intensive phase may improve outcomes.

The main harm of the 8-month retreatment regimen with first-line drugs is that previously treated patients who *do* have MDR (15.3% at the global level) will receive inadequate treatment during the weeks to months of waiting for DST results. Patients may become more ill and wasted, spread MDR-TB to others, and seek care from providers not linked to the NTP who may not follow NTP treatment guidelines. Use of the retreatment first-line drug regimen in MDR patients may also result in acquired ethambutol resistance.

Other considerations

For retreatment patients at medium to low likelihood of MDR, the following alternatives to the first-line drug retreatment regimen were considered and rejected:

- 6HRZE may be effective against isoniazid-resistant *M. tuberculosis* (see Question 3), but toxicity is a concern when pyrazinamide is used throughout therapy.

- 2HRZE/4HRE is recommended for use in new patients with high levels of isoniazid resistance (see Question 3), but 10.3% of previously treated patients have ethambutol resistance (compared with 2.5% of new patients) (4), which would render this regimen less effective.

- Omission of streptomycin from the retreatment regimen was rejected given that this injectable may strengthen this regimen (see Question 3) and does not compromise amikacin or kanamycin for use in MDR patients.

- Using the same 6-month regimen as is used for new patients was also rejected. For the 15.3% of previously treated patients who do have MDR, the 4-month isoniazid and rifampicin continuation phase would theoretically not jeopardize ethambutol to the same extent as the 8-month regimen with its 5HRE continuation phase. For the 12.4% of previously treated patients who have isoniazid resistance but not MDR, the isoniazid and rifampicin continuation phase could lead to acquired MDR. Thus the possible benefit of using the new patient regimen to preserve ethambutol in MDR patients is probably outweighed by the risk of acquiring rifampicin resistance in the scenario of pre-existing isoniazid resistance.

- The option of augmenting the 8-month retreatment regimen with a fluoroquinolone or an injectable other than streptomycin was rejected in order to preserve these two classes of drugs, which form the backbone of MDR-TB treatment.

Conclusion

When compared with the alternative of providing an MDR regimen to all previously treated patients, the risks (toxicity, cost and development of resistance to important MDR drugs) outweigh the benefits. There was no other alternative found to the 8-month retreatment regimen with first-line drugs. Since the evidence for this regimen is of very low quality, this is a conditional recommendation.

■ **Recommendation 7.1**
  Specimens for culture and drug susceptibility testing (DST) should be obtained from all previously treated TB patients at or before the start of treatment. DST should be performed for at least isoniazid and rifampicin

■ **Recommendation 7.2**
  In settings where rapid DST is available, the results should guide the choice of regimen

■ **Recommendation 7.3**
  In settings where rapid DST results are not routinely available to guide the management of individual patients, empirical treatment should be started as follows:

  ■ **Recommendation 7.3.1**
    TB patients whose treatment has *failed* or other patient groups with high likelihood of multidrug-resistant TB (MDR) should be started on an empirical MDR regimen

  ■ **Recommendation 7.3.2**
    TB patients returning after defaulting or relapsing from their first treatment course may receive the retreatment regimen containing first-line drugs 2HRZES/1HRZE/5HRE if country-specific data show low or medium levels of MDR in these patients or if such data are unavailable

■ **Recommendation 7.4**

In settings where DST results are not yet routinely available to guide the management of individual patients, the empirical regimens will continue throughout the course of treatment

■ **Recommendation 7.5**

National TB control programmes (NTPs) should obtain and use their country-specific drug resistance data on failure, relapse and default patient groups to determine the levels of MDR

References

1. Menzies D et al. Effect of duration and intermittency of rifampin on tuberculosis treatment outcomes – a systematic review and meta-analysis. *PloS Medicine*, 2009, 6:e1000146.

2. Jindani A, Nunn AJ, Enarson DA. Two 8-month regimens of chemotherapy for treatment of newly diagnosed pulmonary tuberculosis: international multicentre randomised trial. *Lancet*, 2004, 364:1244–1251.

3. Mitchison DA. Basic mechanisms of chemotherapy. *Chest*, 1979, 76(6 Suppl.): 771–781.

4. *Anti-tuberculosis drug resistance in the world: fourth global report.* Geneva, World Health Organization, 2008 (WHO/HTM/TB/2008.394).

5. Khan FA et al. Treatment of active tuberculosis in HIV co-infected patients: a systematic review and meta-analysis. *Clinical Infectious Diseases*, 2010 (in press).

6. American Thoracic Society, CDC, Infectious Diseases Society of America. Treatment of tuberculosis. *Morbidity and Mortality Weekly Report: Recommendations and Reports*, 2003, 52(RR-11):1–77.

7. Schünemann HJ et al. Grading quality of evidence and strength of recommendations for diagnostic tests and strategies. *British Medical Journal*, 2008, 336:1106–1110.

8. Menzies D et al. Standardized treatment of active tuberculosis in previously treated patients, and/or with mono-resistance to isoniazid – a systematic review and meta-analysis. *PloS Medicine*, 2009, 6:e1000150.

TB treatment outcomes

For the meeting in October 2008, members of the Guidelines Group scored the TB treatment outcomes that they considered to be the most critical for the choice of TB treatment regimens. They were asked to take the point of view of NTP managers – the target audience for this publication. Of the 19 members who attended that meeting, 15 (79%) responded; the results are shown below.

Score   *Relative importance*

1–3   Not important for making recommendations on TB regimen
4–6   Important but not critical for making recommendations on TB regimen
7–9   Critical for making recommendations on TB regimen

What are the most important *beneficial* outcomes to consider when making decisions on TB treatment regimens?

Outcomes	Relative importance
Reducing emergence of MDR-TB, prevent drug resistance	8
Survival	8
Staying disease-free (avoiding relapse)	8
Halting transmission of TB, a TB-free community	8
Bacteriological cure	6
Negative sputum smears at 2 months	6
Relief of TB symptoms	5
Cost savings	5

What are the most significant *risks* to consider when making decisions on TB treatment regimens?

Outcomes	Relative importance
Acquired drug resistance	8
Failure	8
Relapse	8
Infecting health care workers and the community	7
Default	7
Loss of efficacy of HIV medicines due to poorly managed drug interactions	7
Drug toxicity	7
Interaction with non-TB medications	6
Financial burden	5

Implementation and evaluation of the fourth edition

A strategy for effective uptake requires definition of the key messages, the audiences and the actions for them to take. The key messages of this fourth edition are the eight strong recommendations listed in Table A4.1. By designating them as "strong", the Guidelines Group is confident that their implementation will yield significant health benefits, outweighing any potential harms.[1]

Table A4.1 STRONG RECOMMENDATIONS

No.	Recommendation
New patients	
1.1 1.2	Replace 6HE in the continuation phase with 4HR
2.1	Implement daily treatment throughout the course of therapy
2.4	Discontinue regimens using twice weekly dosing throughout therapy
HIV-positive TB patients, whether their TB is new or previously treated	
4.1 4.2	TB patients living with HIV, and all patients living in HIV-prevalent settings, should receive daily TB treatment at least during the intensive phase (optimally, also in the continuation phase)
4.4	For TB patients living with HIV, implement at least the same duration of daily treatment as for HIV-negative patients
Sputum monitoring during TB treatment (new and previously treated)	
5.2	Perform additional sputum examination at month 3 if sputum smear is positive at month 2 (in new patients)
5.3 5.4	Obtain specimen for culture and DST if sputum smear-positive at month 3 (in new and previously treated patients)
Treatment extension	
6	No need for extending the intensive phase of treatment. That recommendation will require changes in training and drug supply systems

Key audiences for these recommendations are members of international TB organizations, WHO regional offices, and national TB control programmes (especially in countries with high TB burdens, high levels of MDR-TB and/or TB/HIV). Target audiences within countries include other TB service providers working in public and

---

[1] Because the rest of the recommendations are conditional, they are lower priority for implementation and evaluation.

private health care facilities at the central and peripheral levels (see section 1.3). The actions for all the target audiences are to implement these eight recommendations in the context of their overall TB priorities.

Monitoring and evaluation should be built into implementation, in order to provide important lessons for uptake and continued implementation (1). In the framework presented in Table A4.2, these eight strong recommendations are *inputs* that should improve the *processes* of TB treatment and reporting, which in turn should improve the *outcomes* of treatment success and reduced drug resistance, and finally have an impact on reducing TB prevalence, incidence and death.

Table A4.2 FRAMEWORK FOR EVALUATING THE IMPACT OF THE FOURTH EDITION[a]

Indicator types	Indicators
Input	Activities (such as NTP manual revised to adopt new recommendations)
Process	Improve TB management (such as proportion of previously treated patients with culture and DST performed on sputum specimens at the start of therapy)
Outcome	Improve treatment success (such as proportion of previously treated patients who are cured)
Impact	Reduce TB prevalence, incidence and death (MDG 6) Reduce poverty (MDG 1)[b]

[a] Adapted from: *DOTS Expansion Working Group Strategic Plan 2006–2015.* Geneva, World Health Organization, 2006 (WHO/HTM/TB?2006.370), p. 6.
[b] MDG = Millennium Development Goal.

Necessary steps for implementation of specific recommendations; corresponding evaluation indicators

The necessary steps (prerequisites) for implementing each recommendation are listed below. For all eight recommendations, information on the following outcome and impact indicators is already routinely collected (or estimated):

- Outcome indicators: cure, treatment success, default (recording and reporting forms, WHO's annual *Global tuberculosis control* report), level of drug resistance (drug resistance surveys).

- Impact indicators: TB incidence and mortality (WHO's *Global tuberculosis control* report (2)).

Specific process indicators for evaluating each recommendation are listed below.

Recommendation 1.1

New patients with pulmonary TB should receive a regimen containing 6 months' rifampicin: 2HRZE/4HR.

Recommendation 1.2

The 2HRZE/6HE treatment regimen should be phased out.

Prerequisites:

- In countries that have been using a self-administered continuation phase, expand supervised treatment to allow rifampicin to be given safely throughout therapy.

Process indicators for evaluation (WHO's *Global tuberculosis control* report (*2*), GDF data):

— number[1] of countries changing to the 4-month isoniazid and rifampicin continuation phase;
— number of new patients receiving the 6 months' rifampicin regimen;
— number of patients with supervised treatment throughout therapy.

Recommendation 2.2

New patients with TB should not receive twice weekly dosing for the full course of treatment unless this is done in the context of formal research.

Recommendation 4.1

TB patients with known positive HIV status and all TB patients living in HIV-prevalent settings should receive daily TB treatment at least during the intensive phase.

Prerequisites:

- Expand treatment supervision in countries that have been using twice weekly dosing for any TB patients, or three times weekly intensive-phase dosing for TB patients who are HIV-positive or living in an HIV-prevalent setting.

Process indicators for evaluation (WHO's *Global tuberculosis control* report (*2*), Global Drug Facility data):

— number of countries eliminating twice weekly dosing schedules;
— number of countries in which NTP guidelines change to recommend daily intensive-phase treatment of HIV-positive TB patients;
— number of HIV-positive patients receiving daily intensive-phase treatment.

Global level actions for implementation and evaluation

At the global level, implementation and evaluation of these eight recommendations will necessitate:

- WHO and partners assisting countries to establish drug resistance surveys of new patients, and ongoing surveillance of DST of all previously treated patients. This will require strengthened laboratory capacity.

---

[1] Other calculations (such as proportions) will also be useful.

- WHO and partners assisting countries to ensure treatment supervision throughout therapy.

- WHO and partners identifying, and assisting in the updating of, existing training materials and other technical tools (such as guidance for Global Fund applications, district and health facility training modules), and fostering their uptake and use.

- WHO updating instructions and forms for recording and reporting and assisting countries with implementation.

- WHO adjusting indicators (3, 4) to capture the data needed to evaluate these recommendations (i.e. proportion of failure, relapse and default patients with culture and DST performed at the start of therapy).

- The Global Drug Facility (GDF) re-forecasting drug needs, providing guidance to countries on the transition from old to new regimens, and proposing a phase-out plan for existing stocks in public and private sectors (5).

- The MDR-TB treatment programmes scaling up (including availability of quality-assured second-line drugs) now that an MDR regimen is recommended as part of each country s standard regimens.

The recommendations in these guidelines support the Global Plan to Stop TB (4) and the Stop TB Strategy (6). Implementation of the four recommendations for *previously treated* patients is already part of the programme of work of the WHO Stop TB Department and the MDR-TB Working Group (MDR-TB WG) of the Stop TB Partnership. The other recommendations represent changes to standardized treatment under the DOTS component of the Global Plan to Stop TB, for which the WHO Stop TB Department – in partnership with the DOTS Expansion Working Group (DEWG) – is responsible. The latter includes the Global Laboratory Initiative (GLI), which is in the process of expanding capacity for culture and DST. The HIV/TB Working Group (TB/HIV WG) could foster implementation of daily intensive-phase dosing for TB patients who are HIV-positive or living in HIV-prevalent settings.

A broad group of stakeholders from NTPs, international organizations providing TB technical assistance (including WHO regional and country offices), members of the WHO Strategic, Technical and Advisory Group (STAG TB), and patient representatives were engaged as members of the Guidelines Group in the development of this fourth edition (Annex 6). The involvement of these members of the target audience throughout the development process should increase buy-in and facilitate implementation. Synchronization of this revision with updates to the *International standards for tuberculosis care* (7) should help pave the way towards adoption by private practitioners working at the country level.

WHO and international partners can incorporate these new recommendations in their ongoing technical support and capacity-building efforts in countries. Existing mechanisms for technical assistance also include TBTEAM, the Green Light Committee (GLC) Initiative, and the GDF. International partners can also help countries to incorporate these recommendations into their country-specific TB plans and to mobilize funding from domestic sources or international financing mechanisms (such as the Global Fund to Fight AIDS, Tuberculosis and Malaria). As the recommendations are implemented, evaluation of a number of indicators is already built in to routine monitoring of progress towards targets and Global Plan implementation.

Additional global level actions could include:

* Develop, budget and implement a communication and dissemination plan including presentations at international meetings and working group meetings.

* Prepare multiple formats (information products) such as:

  — placing the guidelines on the WHO web site;
  — translating into official WHO languages;
  — summary of recommendations;
  — policy briefs for international and country use;
  — inclusion in WHO Technical Report Series indexed on Medline (with ISBN).

* Plan for and assist with regional/country implementation:

  — work with technical partners and with WHO regional and country offices to determine which recommendations are priorities for implementation and evaluation in which regions;
  — analyse capacity of health systems in high-burden countries to adopt and evaluate the new recommendations.

Regional and country level actions

Regions and countries will need to select the recommendations that have the highest priority for implementation in the context of regional and national TB plans, local epidemiology and health systems. For example, introduction of liquid media for culture and DST should be based on comprehensive country-specific plans for laboratory capacity-strengthening. A country with high error rates in smear microscopy will first strengthen external quality assurance of microscopy before introducing culture. Similarly, the recommendations for treatment regimens must be implemented in the context of the country s drug management and supply systems. A country with frequent stock outs of first-line drugs will address this problem before changing continuation phase-drugs to implement Recommendation 1.

Additional country and regional level actions could include:

* Translating the fourth edition into appropriate languages as needed.

* Evaluating surveillance data to target particular countries for implementation and evaluation of specific recommendations. For example, the 2009 WHO *Global*

tuberculosis control report showed that 23 countries were still using the 6HE continuation phase.

- Assisting countries in securing funding for, planning, implementing and evaluating these recommendations.

- Convening stakeholders (including professional associations) to:
  — analyse the need for the change at regional or country level and the risks and benefits of implementing the recommendation;
  — analyse the capacity (public and private sector) of the region or country to implement the change;
  — identify and quantify factors that may constrain or facilitate successful implementation;
  — develop regional or country policy and obtain endorsement.

- Develop a plan for implementation and evaluation, including:
  — key inputs and budget;
  — sequencing of key tasks (which may include a feasibility study or demonstration projects) and how the change will be phased in gradually (or rolled out all at once);
  — training of health workers and community partners, coordinated with supply and infrastructure changes;
  — revision of recording and reporting forms;
  — develop, field test, and disseminate an operational guide and toolkit to assist countries and decision-makers to implement and evaluate the new recommendations.

- Develop a communication plan, including briefing decision-makers in the ministry of health, professional associations, and donors. Ensure consistent messages are communicated to health care workers, community partners providing care, and the public. This could include developing a pocket card and wall poster combining Tables 3.2, 3.3 and 3.4 (to replace categories I–IV). Include names for the "new patient", "retreatment with first-line drugs", and "MDR" regimens to replace the familiar nicknames of the previous treatment scheme: "categories 1, 2", etc.

- Assist national TB control programmes in updating national TB guidelines and manuals, laboratory standard operating procedures, TB section of HIV guidelines, drug supply management systems.

References

1. *New technologies for tuberculosis control: a framework for their adoption, introduction and implementation.* Geneva, World Health Organization, 2007 (WHO/HTM/STB/2007.40).

2. *Anti-tuberculosis drug resistance in the world: fourth global report.* Geneva, World Health Organization, 2008 (WHO/HTM/TB/2008.394).

3. *Monitoring and evaluation toolkit: HIV/AIDS, TB, malaria, and health systems strengthening*, 3rd ed. Geneva, The Global Fund to Fight AIDS, Tuberculosis and Malaria, 2009 (available at http://www.theglobalfund.org).

4. *The Global Plan to Stop TB, 2006–2015.* Geneva, World Health Organization, 2006 (WHO/HTM/STB/2006.35).

5. *Compendium of indicators for monitoring and evaluating national tuberculosis programmes.* Geneva, World Health Organization(WHO/HTM/TB/2004.344; (available at: http://whqlibdoc.who.int/hq/2004/WHO_HTM_TB_2004.344.pdf).

6. Phanouvong S. *Operational guide for national tuberculosis control programmes on the introduction and use of fixed-dose combination drugs.* Geneva, World Health Organization, 2002 (WHO/CDS/TB/2002.308).

7. *International standards for tuberculosis care*, 2nd ed. The Hague, Tuberculosis Coalition for Technical Assistance, 2009.

Suggestions for future research

At many points during the process of revising the third edition, future research needs were identified. There was often no evidence available to allow the formulation of recommendations for specific issues; sometimes the only available evidence was judged to be of low quality. While seven questions are the focus of this fourth edition, additional questions emerged.

Gaps in the evidence and additional questions are summarized below as suggestions for future research. A few may be amenable to systematic reviews, but others will require clinical trials, large cohort studies, epidemiological studies, or behavioural research. The suggestions are listed (in no order of priority) under each of the seven questions.

1. Duration of rifampicin in HIV-negative TB patients

- For various forms of drug resistance (other than MDR), and balanced against tolerability and costs, what is the minimum number of effective drugs for the intensive and continuation phases?

- In particular countries followed prospectively, what is the cost and impact of changing from a 6HE to a 4HR continuation phase?

- In new cases of TB meningitis (and other forms of extrapulmonary TB), what is the optimal duration of treatment?

2. Intermittent dosing

- In new pulmonary TB patients, does daily treatment throughout the course of therapy, compared with a twice weekly or 3 times weekly intermittent regimen throughout the course of therapy, reduce relapse, failure and acquired drug resistance?

- What is the impact of drug resistance on outcomes after intermittent regimens?

- What is the impact on adherence of three times weekly dosing, for example when provided by a family member after a daily intensive phase?

- How important is earlier culture conversion (associated with a daily intensive phase) to patient outcomes and TB transmission?

3. Treatment of new patients where isoniazid resistance is high

- In new patients with smear-positive pulmonary TB, does HRE in the continuation phase for 4 months reduce failure, relapse and acquired drug resistance compared with HR?

- What is the efficacy of ethambutol in preventing acquisition of rifampicin resistance in patients with pretreatment isoniazid resistance?

- What other efficacious and tolerable regimens exist for isoniazid-resistant TB?

- What is the incidence of ocular toxicity due to ethambutol?

- Do new patients with isoniazid resistance respond differently from previously treated patients with the same drug resistance profile?

4. HIV-related TB

- In new HIV-positive patients with smear-positive pulmonary TB who are given ART, does a 9-month rifampicin-based TB treatment regimen, compared with a 6-month rifampicin-based regimen, increase treatment success rate and reduce recurrent TB at the end of treatment and for the first 12 months after successful completion of treatment?

- In patients on ART, what is the impact of three times weekly treatment compared with daily treatment during the continuation phase on mortality, failure, relapse and acquired drug resistance?

5. Sputum monitoring

- Using data from Union Study A and C, determine how well positive bacteriological results at various months of treatment predict failure and relapse, compared with negative bacteriological results.

- Reanalyse data from the British Medical Research Council to study patients who are smear-positive during 2 consecutive months. Of those patients who are smear-positive at 2 months, how many are still smear-positive at 3 months? Of these, how many are culture-positive? What is the ability to predict treatment outcomes? (Repeat with other pairs of months.)

- How well can sputum monitoring predict pretreatment or acquired MDR-TB?

- How useful is the monitoring of smear conversion as an indicator of TB control programme performance?

- How often does persistent smear-positivity at the second month of treatment trigger patient or programmatic interventions?

6. Extension of treatment

- For preventing relapse, which patients stand to benefit most from treatment extension? Other than positive smear microscopy, what risk factors (such as patient weight) predict poor outcomes, and can feasibly be ascertained in resource-limited settings?

- Should the intensive phase or the continuation phase be extended, by how long, and with which drugs?

- In adults with pulmonary TB, does performing smear microscopy at the end of the intensive phase and, if sputum is smear-positive, extending this phase reduce failure, relapse or acquired drug resistance?

7. Previously treated patients

- In new smear-positive pulmonary TB patients who have failed first-line TB treatment does an empirical MDR-TB regimen, compared with the standard WHO retreatment regimen with first-line drugs, increase treatment success rate and reduce failure at the end of this second course of TB treatment?

- What is the level of MDR in subgroups of previously treated patients (failed first vs. subsequent course of therapy; returned after defaulting; relapsed)?

Members of the Guidelines Group (Technical Development Group)

Solange Cavalcante
TB Control Program Coordinator, Rio de Janeiro Municipality, Almirante Alexandrino 3780 Bloco E3 302, Santa Tereza cep, 20241-262 – Rio de Janeiro, RJ, Brazil

Jeremiah Muhwa Chakaya (Chairperson)
Technical Expert, National Leprosy and TB Programme, Kenya Medical Research Institute, PO Box 20781, 00202 Nairobi, Kenya

Saidi M. Egwaga
Programme Manager, National TB and Leprosy Programme, Ministry of Health and Social Welfare, P.O. Box 9083, Dar es Salaam, United Republic of Tanzania

Robert Gie
Professor of Medicine, Department of Paediatrics & Child Health, University of Stellenbosch, Faculty of Medicine, PO Box 19063, 7505 Tygerberg, South Africa

Peter Gondrie
Executive Director, KNCV Tuberculosis Foundation, PO Box 146, Parkstraat 17 (Hofstaete Building), 2501 CC The Hague, Netherlands

Anthony D. Harries
Senior Consultant, International Union Against Tuberculosis and Lung Disease, Old Inn Cottage, Vears Lane, Colden Common, Winchester, Hants, England

Phillip Hopewell
Professor of Medicine, Division of Pulmonary & Critical Care, San Francisco General Hospital, Building NH, SFGH Rm 5H5, University of California San Francisco (UCSF), San Francisco, CA 94143-0841, USA

Blessina Kumar
Flat B-13, Lakeview Apartment, Plot 886, Ward 8, Mehrauli, New Delhi 110030, India

Kitty Lambregts-van Weezenbeek
Senior Consultant, KNCV Tuberculosis Foundation, PO Box 146, Parkstraat 17 (Hofstaete Building), 2501 CC The Hague, Netherlands

Sundari Mase
Division of TB Elimination National Centre for HIV, STD and TB, Centers for Disease Control and Prevention, 1600 Clifton Road NE, MS E-10 Corporate Square Building, Bldg 10, Atlanta, GA 30333, USA

Richard Menzies
Director, Respiratory Division, MUHC and McGill University, Room K1.24, Montreal Chest Institute, 3650 St Urbain Street, Montreal, PQ, Canada

Anna Nakanwagi Mukwaya
Chief of Party, TBCAP Program, International Union Against Tuberculosis and Lung Disease, Plot 2 Loudel Road, Nakasero, PO BOX 16094, Wandegeya, Uganda

Mahshid Nasehi
National TB Programme Manager, Centre for Disease Control & Prevention, Ministry of Health and Medical Education, 68 Iranshahr Street, Ferdowsi Square, 11344 Tehran, Islamic Republic of Iran

Andrew Nunn
Professor of Epidemiology, Associate Director, MRC Clinical Trials Unit, 222 Euston Road, London NW1 2DA, England

Madhukar Pai
Assistant Professor, Department of Epidemiology, Biostatistics & Occupational Health, McGill University, 1020 Pine Avenue West, Montreal, PQ H3A 1A2, Canada

Holger Schünemann
Methodologist, Chair, McMaster University Medical Centre, Clinical Epidemiology and Biostatistics, Health Sciences Centre 2C10B, 1200 W. Main Street, Hamilton, ON L8N 3Z5, Canada

Zarir F. Udwadia
Private Practitioner and Consultant Physician, Hinduja Hospital and Research Centre, Mumbai, India

Andrew Vernon
Division of TB Elimination, National Centre for HIV, STD and TB, Centers for Disease Control and Prevention, 1600 Clifton Road NE, MS E-10 Corporate Square Building, Building 10, Atlanta, GA 30333, USA

Rozalind G. Vianzon
National TB Programme Manager, National Center for Disease Control and Prevention, Department of Health, 4th Floor, Building 13, San Lazaro Compound, Santa Cruz, Manila, Philippines

Virginia Williams
TB Project Director, International Council of Nurses, Gardeners Barn, Cock Road, Eye, Suffolk IP23 7NS, England

External Review Group

Olayide Akanni, Nigeria
Margareth Pretti Dalcolmo, Brazil
Francis Drobniewski, United Kingdom
Paula Fujiwara, USA
Salmaan Keshavjee, USA
G.R. Khatri, India
Michail Perelman, Russian Federation
Charles Sandy, Zimbabwe
Pedro Guillermo Suarez, Peru
Marieke van der Werf, Netherlands
Wang Lixia, China
Nadia Wiweko, Indonesia

Mohamed Abdel Aziz, The Global Fund to Fight AIDS, Tuberculosis and Malaria
Daniel Kibuga, WHO Regional Office for Africa
Giampaolo Mezzabotta, WHO Viet Nam
Jamhoih Tonsing, Family Health International Cambodia
Richard Zaleskis, WHO Regional Office for Europe